NATURE CURE

(FORMERLY CALLED WATER CURE)

or

Home Treatment without Medicine

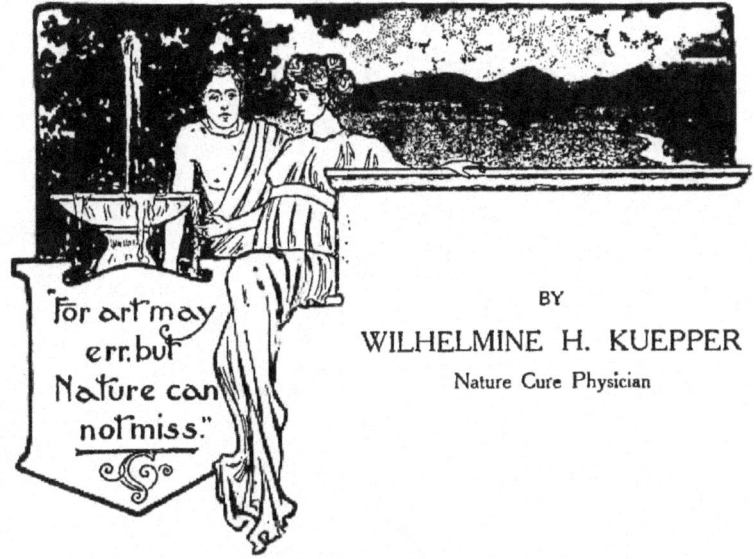

"For art may err, but Nature can not miss."

BY

WILHELMINE H. KUEPPER

Nature Cure Physician

"Better be unborn than untaught; for ignorance is the root of misfortune."—*Plato.*

THE JOHN C. WINSTON COMPANY

PHILADELPHIA

CHICAGO   TORONTO

1905

ERRATA

PAGE 106.—Omit reference to Fig. 21 in foot note.

PAGES 160 AND 185.—Omit reference to Fig. 18 in foot note.

PAGE 189.—For Fig. 26 read Fig. 25, and for Fig. 25 read 26.

PAGE 191.—For Fig. 21 read Fig. 17.

PART I.

NATURE CURE AND MEDICINE.

PART II.

DISEASES TREATED.

NATURE CURE

OR

Home Treatment Without Medicine

CONTENTS.

PART I.

NATURE CURE AND MEDICINE.

PART II.

DISEASES TREATED.

PART III.

TREATMENTS EXPLAINED.

PART IV.

HYGIENIC COOKING.

RECIPES.

.

INTRODUCTION

"The most precious possession of a country and society is man. Every life represents a certain value. To keep it intact to its end is not only humane, but in their own interest, the duty of any Commonwealth."—*Prince Rudolf of Austria.*

"Follow Nature; she is the best teacher, and makes never a mistake."—*Pestalozzy.*

THE very best thing man can possess is health, and wise are they who strive to regain and keep it.

A great reform movement in medicine is going on now. It is gaining daily, and the "thinking" people of our time see its need.

To supply this need there has appeared quite a number of "cures" or healing methods; for, what the people want, ever so many endeavor to provide. Nature Cure, formerly called "Water Cure," though, crowns all other methods. It gives to our bodies what Nature herself uses in creating and maintaining a healthy physique—air, light, sun, water, wholesome food, to which we add proper dress, dwellings, exercise and rest, according to need, and with massage as a substitute for exercise, and as a healing factor in many chronic diseases.

For more than fifty years in Germany it has had

a hard fight against medicine, but now it is more and
more recognized there, and forms part of the curri-
culum in some of their medical universities. In the
United States quite a number of Nature Cure Sanitariums have been established and flourish, among
others the Battle Creek Sanitarium, in Battle Creek,
Mich.; Dr. Carl Strueh's Sanitarium, Chicago; Sanitarium Jungborn, at Bellevue, Butler, N. Y.; Dr.
Sheppard's, 81 Columbia Heights, Brooklyn, N. Y.,
and many others. Let us follow their example by
spreading it for the benefit of suffering humanity,
and by helping to bring up a healthier generation.

How soon we lose respect for a man who professes
to know that with which he is not conversant, or to
be that which he is not. No business man can long
keep our confidence if he prove ignorant of the
principles of his work. To-day we find, more than
ever, schools for training our young people for the
various walks of life, and for rendering them more
fit to be good and able citizens.

If this is so necessary elsewhere, why should not
the future parents of the land receive some instruction as to the duties of their high and holy calling?
Do we value the physical body so lightly that we can
afford to remain in ignorance of its most funda-
mental hygienic laws?

Surely not. Then why should not our young men
and women be most carefully instructed in the duties
of fatherhood and motherhood? Why should they
be allowed to enter into that most sacred of relation-
ships more ignorant than even the lower animals?

These, by nature, are protected to a degree through their instinct, a power almost, if not wholly, lost to man, through centuries of wrong living. If reforms are ever necessary—if society, or the human race, is to be radically benefited, here we must begin, and our young people must be taught that their physical bodies are the "Temples of the Lord," and to use them and respect them as such. If this book helps some to such an uplifting of their ideas, and so results in some happy homes, where disease, with its train of evils, is properly met and naturally defeated, the writer will feel that her life has not been in vain.

We want to feel, with the great poet, that

> "All are but parts of one stupendous whole
> Whose body Nature is, and God the soul."

Marriage, as we all know, is fundamentally for the reproduction of the race. "Multiply and replenish the earth" is a Divine command, which lays upon us a duty, and those who enter into married life and undertake the fulfilment of this command should see to it that they fulfill not only the letter but the spirit of the law, and so produce only healthy offspring. To do otherwise is a crime. Sickly, ailing weaklings have no cause to be grateful to those who gave them life. Far from it, they will curse them for their misery, and as the sins of the fathers were visited on them, so by their example they, in turn, do likewise; and thus it happens that every generation grows weaker, and that it is rare, even now, to find a person with a perfect physique. This must stop, and everyone should do his part in this reform.

How can we stop it? By learning on what our health depends. It depends upon the natural life—factors common to all creatures—air, light, water, food and drink, exercise and rest. To those must be added proper clothing, dwelling, etc. If these life-factors are natural to us, then the conditions of health are fulfilled; otherwise we shall grow sick.

What is sickness? It is an incomplete change of matter in our bodies, caused by a wrong way of living. In olden times most people were strong and healthy, and the weak and sickly were despised. They were strong because they lived close to Nature and did not take any medicine. Imagine Adam and Eve taking medicine!

Man has strayed away from Nature, and the punishment is disease. Let us go back to Nature, and in order to do this let us take for our example the large animals of the lower order. They are out-of-doors in all kinds of weather, summer and winter. As few of us can be out-of-doors all the time, let us do the next best thing—sleep with open windows, and take out-of-door exercise as much as possible; walk to our business, instead of riding in close cars filled with bad air, and ventilate well our offices, workshops, schoolrooms, etc.

Our skin is an excreting and breathing organ, therefore it ought to come in contact with the air. But most people wear so much clothing, tightly woven, that it is impossible for the skin to act well; and as the skin is doing incomplete work, the balance which it does not do falls on the inner organs—lungs, kidneys, liver, bowels, etc. As many organs are not strong enough to do this double work for years and years they finally give out, and serious disturbances follow. Therefore take air baths at least every morning and evening, and do not overdress.

Air is more important to us than food, because we can live without the latter for weeks, but not an hour without air. Our dwellings should be dry, sunny and well ventilated.

After you have grown strong through a hygienic way of living, enter into married life—not frivolously and imprudently, for it is the most important step in life. Make the union only with a healthy partner, and let your physician inform and advise you about everything you ought to know concerning this new phase of life.

This book is intended to instruct its readers how to live in order to produce a healthier generation, and how to help themselves when sick. We shall aim to explain the different forms of treatment, so that they will be thoroughly understood and successfully applied. As it is richly illustrated, there ought to be no difficulty in understanding its explanations.

My esteemed teacher, Dr. Max Boehm, has kindly permitted me to use his book, and to select quotations from it, for which special favor I owe him many thanks.

In order to do your part in helping mankind, follow the Doctor's advice: "Give every bride friend a book of natural hygiene; teach all children in school how to live right; make them hygienists of their own bodies, and the future happiness of mankind is assured.''

This book will supply a much-felt want; it will teach you to become your own physician, as everybody naturally ought to be. And after you are well it will teach you how to live in order never to grow sick again, for sickness is punishment for a wrong way of living. We ought to be well and die of old age *without disease,* like the animals in their natural state. ''Nature Cure'' ought to be in every house, for although when sick you may call in a physician, there are many instances where relief from pain, health, and even life, depends on quick action before the doctor can arrive; for instance, in hemorrhages, poisoning, burns, wounds, hydrophobia, infantile paralysis, sprained ankle, fainting, epilepsy, broken bones, concussion of the brain, besides those sudden painful attacks which almost always come during the night—gout, whooping cough, asthma, colic, etc., etc. You will feel so much more happy knowing if any of these attacks should befall one of your dear ones that you could give effectual help.

And you will save the cost of the book a hundredfold if you only follow its directions in one case of sickness, being convinced at the same time that Nature Cure treatment cannot do any harm to the patient, but will improve him with every application.

All physicians and nurses ought to have it, for they more than anybody ought to advance with the most important science in the world, physical dietetic therapy, which recently has made and is making such great strides.

Medical science has searched in vain for thousands of years for means to conquer and abolish disease, but with the increase of medicines the diseases have increased instead of diminishing. The vitality of our own body is the main curative power in the world, which we have only to direct and to assist when it is weak.

WILHELMINE H. KUEPPER.

Germantown, Philadelphia, Pa.

PART I.

NATURE CURE AND MEDICINE

First follow Nature, and your judgment frame
By her just standard, which is still the same;
Unerring Nature, still divinely bright;
One clear, unchanged, and universal light,
Life, Force, and Beauty, must to all impart,
At once the source, and end, and test of art.—*Pope.*

DURING the past century great advancement in natural sciences and in medicine has been made. The advancement in medicine has kept pace with that of all other sciences, except in one department, therapeutics. By this we do not mean to say that therapeutics was not or is not advancing, but that the advancement is due, not to what is commonly understood as medical science, but to the development of Nature Cure science. This progress, therefore, is not along the old beaten paths of pharmacology, but by what we may call physical dietetic therapy. We shall try to show the difference between the therapeutics as developed by Nature Cure science and the therapeutics of regular medicine, which difference is of vital importance. Since the body is an organism possessing natural healing powers, Nature Cure treats the ailments more in a general way than locally. The aim of

15

Nature Cure is to conquer the cause of the disease, not merely to suppress the symptoms.

Nature Cure applies natural healing factors rather than foreign substances, such as medicines. The body is not a conglomeration of single parts—heart, lungs, liver, etc.—put into a box or frame. It is an organism where the whole works for the existence of the parts, and *vice versa,* and where the principle of compensation is shown to a high degree.

All parts are closely united by the blood-vessels, lymphatics and nerves; therefore anything which disturbs or impairs a single organ affects the whole body, and the body endeavors to resist and throw off anything injurious to any one part of it. This process we call natural healing power. This is easily proved by such physiological phenomena as when a bone is broken, directly this healing power sends a cement (callus) to the place of fracture to unite the ends, and then sets diligently to work to build up tissue and the healing process is complete. A bleeding takes place from a wound. What does this healing power do? It stops the flow by coagulating the blood. If something is eaten which cannot be digested, or which upon entering the blood would harm the body (as in the case of poisoning); this natural healing power tries to expel it by vomiting and by diarrhœa. When a blood-vessel is destroyed by a wound, then the smaller blood-vessels, capillaries, in the locality, which are connected with this blood-vessel, enlarge to sufficiently provide that part of the body with blood (collateral circulation).

When one kidney is unable to act, then the other kidney enlarges and does double duty. In cases where one ventricle of the heart, because of a diseased condition of the valves, has an abnormal amount of work to do, it enlarges to meet the extra demand. When by disease of the lungs, tuberculosis, etc., the upper parts cannot expand enough, the lower parts expand the more in order to take in the necessary amount of oxygen (vicarious emphysema, i. e., one for another).

These are only simple examples, but this natural healing power is just as active in the most complicated diseases and in the highest functions of the body. Usually diseased organs are treated locally by medicines or applications. For instance, in paralysis, an ice-bag on the head; for headache, electric current directly through the head; in stomach troubles, medicines which work directly on this organ; in inflammation of the mucous membrane of the uterus, curetting and cauterizing; in throat diseases, gargling and cauterizing. In diphtheria it was some time ago customary to destroy the coating by cauterizing with nitrate of silver or carbolic acid, by which method sore places were not to be avoided, this only causing the disease to spread. This dangerous practice was recognized by the allopaths themselves, and is now entirely abandoned in Germany. By such local treatment the diseased organ is irritated still more, and eventually overworked by the extra task of expelling the morbid matter. Such a practice seems in the light of our present development crude

2

and mechanical. Nature Cure teaches us to spare the diseased organ as much as possible, and following the above-mentioned indications of Nature to work directly through the regulation of the circulation, increasing the excretions and the change of matter. So we should for a headache apply electricity to the neck and forearms; for inflammation of the throat, a derivative massage, foot packs, foot steams, etc. The single treatment must be adapted to the case, so that under some circumstances a local treatment may properly be applied as well as the general—for instance, a nasal spray, Thure Brandt massage, etc. We may regard many symptoms of disease as an evidence of the natural healing power to expel injurious matter. Nature Cure tries to remove the cause of disease, through which proceeding the symptoms disappear. We can see this best in an example. A patient who, owing to his occupation, is forced to remain in a sitting position all day, eats the average boarding-house diet of much meat and eggs, in consequence of which he soon visits his physician, complaining of headache, cold feet, loss of appetite, constipation, piles, and all the signs of a bad circulation, congestion of the liver and disturbances of the portal circulation produced by the above unwholesome way of living. The regular practitioner will probably give him consecutively a special medicine for each symptom—one for headache, one for constipation and another to create an artificial appetite, while if the piles are large enough he may advise an operation. In consequence of this treatment the patient will have a few days' diminution of his complaint; but the relief does not last long if the sedentary occupation is resumed and the patient continues his diet, which overcharges his digestive organs. Consequently the same symptoms return, since the cause has not been removed. Nature Cure, instead of this symptomatic treatment, would proceed mainly thus (special treatment being naturally adapted to the individual case): Regulation of the circulation by general massage, hot foot-baths, foot steams, drawing the blood from the abdomen by breathing exercises and other gymnastics, advising the patient to counteract the sedentary life which his occupation may demand by exercise in the open air. His diet should contain very little meat, but a great deal of fruit, green vegetables, rice, salads, and his drinks—if he must drink—should consist of lemonade or buttermilk. In this way the injurious influences will be removed and the bad symptoms disappear permanently. On the same principle it is not advisable to stop the symptoms of diarrhœa by opium, as the intestines use this means to cleanse the body from impure matter. Nor is it advisable to give opium indiscriminately to relieve pain. (Nature Cure can in most cases do the same thing by derivative treatment or by the use of cold or steam compresses, etc.) It is the practice of many physicians to remove immediately all that is not quite normal, which is quite contrary to the natural healing power. For instance, it is impossible to check at once a gonorrhœa by injections of sulphate of zinc, nitrate of silver, tannic acid, bichloride of mercury, protargol, resarcin, etc. The great number of these remedies prove their inefficiency. The discharge may be suppressed by them for a while, but sooner or later the patient will have an inflammation of the upper part of the urethra, catarrh of the neck of the bladder, inflammation of the prostate or of the loose connective tissues of the perineum. In short, he will have all the symptoms of a chronic gonorrhœa with all the innumerable sufferings. For the same reasons it would be unwise to suppress or remove all eruptions very quickly, because they are a process of excretion, and ought to be recognized as an endeavor of the natural healing power to expel poison.

For a woman suffering from insomnia, narcotics such as hydrate of chloral may produce drowsiness for a night without removing the cause of the sleeplessness, so that she must take any drug in increasing doses, in order to find out in the end that she has nervous prostration. If we take the trouble to inquire into her way of living, we find that she takes strong coffee in the morning, beefsteak and tea for supper, goes into society, to the theatre and concerts, after which she eats again, and goes to bed after midnight. By simply changing the mode of life of such a patient she would in a very short time enjoy natural sleep, and thus greatly strengthen her nervous system.

Coughing is a reflex action to expel irritating mucus, caused by hypersecretion of an inflamed mucous membrane. If we weaken this action by drugs we work against Nature and retard the cure.

We have mentioned above the compensatory ability of the organs. One often observes, especially in children during the disturbances of the bowels, eruptions of the skin, showing how closely bowels and skin are in sympathy. Thus we can also understand that one can influence skin diseases by regulating the actions of the bowels and by dieting, and indeed we often see that eruptions which have long been treated unsuccessfully by salves, and only suppressed temporarily, are permanently cured by Nature Cure treatment.

Let us now consider fever from this standpoint. Fever is a combination of disturbances in the body, an increase in the change of matter, an abnormal condition of the skin. These symptoms may be caused by disturbances in the central nervous system. It is, therefore, not simply the rise in temperature which measures the degree of fever. Fever is usually regarded as something harmful to the body, a disease in itself, and therefore to be suppressed. Nature Cure regards it as a reaction of the body to overcome the disease, as a natural endeavor of the healing power to expel morbid matter. This increased change of matter is, therefore, the primary symptom which causes the secondary, the increased production of heat. Thus we are led to conclude that in acute infectious diseases the fever must be considered as the consequence of an invasion of foreign living cells entering into a struggle for life with the cells of the tissues. The fever takes place for the preservation of the latter and the destruction of the former. The following observations lead us to such

a theory: We know that the microbes, spirilli of re-
lapsing fever, or typhus recurrence, disappear after
the attack of fever. The attacks of fever of the
various types of malaria are caused also by the increase of the malaria germs (sporalatio of the malaria plasmodium). According to our theory, one
would infer that the degree of fever would corre-
spond to the seriousness of the disease, which, however, is not always the case, for we often see in a low
temperature a fatal end, as in diphtheria, sepsis or
meningitis.

These inferences, however, would be correct if all
people were alike. But how different we are in constitution, development and mode of living! Each has
his *locus minoris resistentiæ.* One has a greater resistive power than another. In one case a good reaction overcomes the illness quickly with powerful
symptoms; in another case the reaction is too weak to
show itself, or the enemy is from the beginning so
strong that all resistance is useless. Strong men
often overcome small disturbances without fever,
while in weak women and children the organism
needs quicker action, fever. In fever the skin is dry;
the secretion of perspiration, the natural compensation of an increased production of heat, is checked.
In many cases we see that after profuse perspiration,
steam baths or bed steam baths, packs work better
here than the antipyretics, which produce perspiration in the beginning by enlarging the vessels of the
skin; but they have their point of attack in the center
of the nervous system, while by the means of Nature

Cure the reflex action, perspiration, is reawakened. On the other hand, it may happen that the natural healing power of the body may be too powerful, as shown in the extremely high temperatures, which in themselves may become alarming. In this case Nature Cure asserts itself, and it also lowers the temperature with surer and less dangerous means, such as sponge baths, quickly changed packs or baths of decreasing temperature. Such means of treatment have the invaluable advantage of decreasing the fever, reviving the strength of the heart, improving the respiration and calming the nervous system. On this account many practitioners of medicine have accepted our treatment for typhoid fever. Many cases of pneumonia end fatally through weakness of the heart, and in typhoid fever through the secondary hypostatic-pneumonia, and it is just in these cases that Nature Cure has gained her first and greatest triumphs. (In many cases the natural healing power is weak, either because it was so from the beginning or because exhausted from many vain efforts to conquer the disease.)

Hippocrates of old declared fever to be a splendid healing power. Professor Harless, of Bonn, said, "Give me the power to create fever and I will cure any disease." Nature Cure can create a kind of artificial fever which it can measure by degrees and stop at will, by various steam applications, sun baths, dry diet, etc. Thus we have seen that in all cases, as well as in fever, it is the duty of the physician to regulate the action of the natural healing power and direct it into the right channels and not to suppress it, for which just as much physiological and medical knowledge is necessary as for the writing of a prescription. The natural, physiological, dietetic healing factors are air, light, water, warmth, cold, rest, motion and diet, as opposed to drugs. Why are the above healing factors called natural ones? Because they are derived from the structure and function of the body. According to the law of preservation of strength and matter, physical and vital powers are most closely connected. Water, air, light, warmth, etc., are for a healthy organism indispensable necessities. Should they not be fit also in a methodical, well-regulated way, artificially applied, to influence the sick organism favorably?

These factors are then a related, adequate stimulation to the cells and are not foreign. What effect these factors have on the organism we see that by the deviation of their normal action, health and life are endangered. All these healing factors such as light, air, sun baths, steam baths, packs, massage and Swedish movements, proper diet and water applications, in their manifold forms, may be exactly individualized, their effect measured and have no injurious secondary effects. This cannot be said of drugs. It is clearly proved by experiments that certain chemical compositions have a certain effect upon the body. For instance, atropin enlarges the pupil of the eye and increases the number of heart beats; brom. potasi. reduces the reflex excitation of the brain, while strychnine increases that of the spinal cord; digitalis reduces and regulates the heart beats, increasing at the same time the pressure of the blood; quicksilver alters the change of matter, namely, it prevents the emigration of the white corpuscles, thus preventing inflammation, and antimony causes vomiting. There are quite a list of medicines which cause diarrhœa, partly by producing vehement motions of the intestines, partly by causing diffusions of serum into the intestines. There are also medicines to produce perspiration. Others reduce the temperature. In this way it is possible for medicines to suppress certain symptoms of disease and cause a temporary relief (let alone those harmful accessory effects connected with them), but they do not cure. First, not in the sense of specifics; there are no specifics. It is against the law of nature to demand for each single disease a specific remedy like poison and anti-poison. It is a vain effort of therapy to find specifica. It will never succeed, in spite of its scientific investigation, because it is against Nature and against the nature of disease.

Disease should be regarded as a disturbance of functions which can be conquered only by helping the organism to re-establish normal conditions through application and regulation of those stimulants which keep up the functions of normal organism. It is just the symptomatical treatment of medicine which proves that the medicines given do not work as specifica. So called, in the sense of medicine, there are only three—quinine for malaria; salicylic acid for acute inflammatory rheumatism, and quicksilver for syphilis. Quinine has a decided influence on the fever attacks of malaria. Sometimes the swollen joints of rheumatism decrease through the use of salicylic acid, and syphilitic symptoms disappear through the use of mercury. But, in spite of all this, they are not specifica. They work only temporarily and symptomatically. This is proved first by the facts observed by every physician, that in many cases they have no effect, and second that, in spite of their use, a relapse and a secondary disease occurs. However great the success of bacteriology, however proud medical science may be of it, little has up to this time resulted from it for therapy. It will always remain a vain effort to kill microbes after they have entered the body and begun to multiply there except the remedies were introduced in such amount or concentrated form as to destroy also the cells of the body. Thus it has been unsuccessful, and it will always remain difficult to kill, for instance, tubercle-bacillus by the aid of chemical means or through inhalations. In all the various treatments of tuberculosis, one has always come to the same result. This was also the final decision of the Berlin Tuberculosis Congress about twenty months ago. Nature Cure brings the patient into the most favorable conditions of life, nourishing diet, fresh air, etc., and makes thus the organism able to resist the intruded enemy.

Even on the exterior, surgery, for good reasons, has replaced the antisepsis by asepsis. One ought to choose by internal diseases rather a "natural asepsis." The effect of medical remedies is not sufficiently understood. A single glance into the history of medicine is sufficient to prove this. The first knowledge of medicine is but rough empiricism.

Even to-day the *post hoc, ergo propter hoc* plays a great rôle, we are sorry to say. Later, from the beginning of the sixteenth century, when medical systems prevailed at certain periods and led to one-sided false ideas, the founders of those 878 terms chose and brought into use those medicines which suited their pathological theories. When in the past century experimental work gained firm ground in the realm of physiology and pathology, pharmacology also began experimenting in order to find out the qualities and effects of all drugs in the most simple and uniform circumstances. But those results gained by experiments on animals cannot be applied indiscriminately to man. It is wrong to compare a pound of cat or dog to a pound of man. Just as daring to adopt the final experiments made on a well person to an ill one. The much affected and partially degenerated heart muscle of a person ill with typhoid fever or tuberculosis reacts from stimulants in a manner different from that of a person in health. Experimenting on patients is even more risky, and oftentimes the drugs most used are the least understood. According to the authorities, morphine is said to produce sleep through contraction of the blood-vessels of the brain. Recently, others think it produces a direct effect on the nervous system.

We do not know whether quinine, which kills microbes outside of the body, will, when administered, just as well directly kill the germs of disease and

malaria within the body, or whether it changes only
the nutritive soil, that is, human protoplasm. The
"how" is not clear. We could mention nearly all the
most-used drugs. If these old, "well-tested" drugs
are but so little understood in their effects, what
about those that change continually, like fashion,
patent medicine, etc., daily brought into the market
by factories? Often the chemical composition of
these preparations is scarcely known, and much
less is the physiological effect tested. If each of these
so much praised remedies is so good and specific a
cure for different diseases, why do they disappear so
quickly from the market to make room for new ones?
The fact that the effects of most drugs, as we have
seen, is not sufficiently known and explained makes it
further clear that they often show besides the intended symptomatic effect a succession of incalcula-
bly harmful secondary effects, so that the devil is
driven out by "Beelzebub, the chief of devils." A
troublesome symptom of a disease may have disappeared through medicine, but in its place several disagreeable medical symptoms have appeared, which
are nothing else than more or less serious symptoms
of poisoning, sometimes injuring the organism permanently.

The singing noticed in the ears and quinine in-
toxication, after large doses of quinine, is well
known. Even after the use of two or three grammes
of salicylic acid, roaring in the ears, deafness and
sometimes vomiting and urticaria show themselves.
In acute rheumatism it is given in doses up to ten

grammes within twenty-four hours; we need not be surprised to see secondary effects, such as great disturbances of digestion, lasting deafness, asthma and mental excitement. The continued use of brom. causes cutaneous eruptions, indigestion, heart affection, trembling of muscles, mental depression and weakness of memory. After a continued use of sulfonal appears weakness of the muscles and often nephritis and destruction of the red corpuscles of the blood.

Often many people suffering from stomach trouble or locomotor ataxia, who were treated with nitrate of silver, show during the rest of their lives a steel gray discoloration of the whole skin. Some physicians deny a third stage of syphilis, and bring the serious bone and nervous diseases of old syphilitics into original connection with former mercurial treatment. However, it is certain that part of the quicksilver given is retained in the body for a longer time. Even if in our day quicksilver is not given in such amounts that the patient, as in former times, starves from mercurial ulcers and necrosis of the jaw, it is practically well known to every physician of to-day that the use of quicksilver causes very often an inflammation of the mouth. Serious irritations of the kidneys appear through the use of cantharides and chloride of potash. After the use of balsam of copaiba, turpentine and sandalwood oil one soon notices loss of appetite, belching, vomiting, diarrhœa, eczema, sometimes albuminuria and hæmaturia. From the use of antifibrin one has to reckon on seri-

ous secondary effects. Besides vomiting and rash
there appear stupor and cyanosis, sometimes swelling
of the liver, uterus and, after continued use, anæmia.
One might go through all the drugs and would
scarcely find one without injurious secondary effects.
Secondary effects of drugs do not appear in all individuals in the same way, nor after the same amount,
for this depends on the sensibility of the organism
and the personal susceptibility to a certain poison.
Here we touch our point, viz., that the effect of medicine individually is very different. Every physician
has had patients with a so-called idiosyncrasy. We
understand by this why some individuals cannot
stand certain drugs, even in a quantity from which
injurious after-effects are not to be anticipated. It is
the same with foods. Some people cannot eat strawberries or oysters, or even smell them, without having
a rash or vomiting. Experience teaches us further
that the same remedy works very differently in children, adults and old people.

It is well known that the use of certain drugs in
childhood is entirely to be avoided, or given with the
greatest precaution.

Manifold modifications in the effects of drugs are
conditioned by habit, way of living, sex, constitution,
temperament and, above all, by the patient's condition. The living body is not a passive, stable machine which is constantly changed by outside influences.

The same substance can sometimes become a remedy and sometimes a poison. There is really between

medicine and poison not a difference in principle, but in degree. We will pass over those cases where patients become morphine habitués through the use of morphine. The inefficiency and dangers of medical therapy being recognized have led to the so-called "nihilismus" in therapy, to the expectative method. This method would only be justified if we had not a better therapy than the medical one, which we have in the physical, dietetic, healing factors. Why, then, wait in expectation, while we could help the patient with these healing factors? Why wait until a more serious or organic disease has developed when we could avoid these through proper treatment of slighter indispositions or functional disturbances? But Nature Cure goes a step farther. Why first lead an unnatural life, which weakens the body and makes it susceptible to diseases, by improper diet, dress, pleasure, work, etc., when one can harden the body and increase its power of resistance by a natural hygienic way of living? Nature Cure teaches a natural prophylaxis and hygiene, and this is her final aim.

In short: Nature Cure is the renaissance of the old humoral therapy, which preceded the era of medicine. The adherents of this method believed that impurities in the fluids of the body were the cause of all diseases. This therapy is proved by the greatest scientists of Germany in our day. Why, Nature herself proves it to us beyond a doubt. For, is not the greatest danger of the disease over, the patient better, and the physician more hopeful when the natural healing power in the patient's body throws out poison in the form of perspiration, boils, rash, diarrhœa, dark urine, etc. The greater the quantity excreted the more rapid will be the patient's recovery.

Nature Cure helps this effort of Nature by producing perspiration, by massage, proper diet, exercise, etc., instead of putting more poisons (drugs) into the diseased body.

HYDROPATHY.

Till taught by pain,
Men really know not what good water's worth;
If you had been in Turkey or in Spain,
Or with a famish'd boat's crew had your berth,
Or in the desert heard the camel's bell,
You'd wish yourself where Truth is—in a well.—*Byron.*

SINCE the creation of the universe water has been the greatest healing factor. We find the proof of this in innumerable quotations from the oldest writings we possess, the Bible not excepted. Hippocrates, the "Father of Medicine," used it frequently, and so did Ambroise Paré, Macartney Sancussani, Caldani, Percy, Surrey, Trall, Priessnitz, Schroth, Rausse, Hahn, Kneipp, in fevers, inflammations, rheumatism, gout, etc., and so did the most renowned physicians up to the present day. Asklepiades, Oribasius, Detius Rhazes, Claicema, Flayer, Haller, Drs. Hoffmann, Gregory, Cheyne, Harvey, Fallopius, Kern, M. Jose of Amiens, Giunninni, Jackson, Forbes, Thaer, Currie, Wright and thousands of renowned physicians of our day and age.

The main portion of our body is water, which is necessary for its existence, for without it bodily combustion would prove fatal.

We use it in various forms, as baths, vapor, packs, pours, enemas, compresses, fomentations, snow, ice.

In its different forms it is cooling, refreshing,

8   33

soothing, quieting; it causes solution and removes impurities. A skin that has been inactive for years can be brought to action and excretion by producing perspiration through the millions of pores on the body by a hot bath and dry pack, and the variously tempered baths not only increase the vitality of the blood and nerves, but help the whole organism.

Most acute diseases can be cured by the well-directed baths and packs in a very short time. A plain lukewarm bath (90° F.) or a cold sponge bath will bring down the fever, as a rule, from one to three degrees, in almost all acute diseases.

In cases of frozen limbs and chilblains, the walking in or rubbing with snow is the most effective cure, followed by scientific massage. For ulcers, small-pox, continued compresses day and night, combined with a fruit diet, will effect a complete cure and prevent scars. For a sore throat, put a fourfold wet cloth, covered with a broader strip of wool Jersey or flannel, around the throat at night. Keep it on all night, and in the morning take it off and wash the throat with cold water.

The headache and toothache often can be cured by a hot foot-bath. A warm bath at night produces sleep, especially when followed by massage.

The various nerve packs are wonderful in their effects; everybody ought to know how to apply them. So are the lung packs for pleurisy, pneumonia, and all lung troubles, etc. In typhoid fever the trunk packs and enemas prevent perforation and purify the system from its poisonous matter, causing a prompt recovery. Every mother ought to know this and teach it to her children. What a help for her to know such simple means of cure, especially if suddenly in the night one of the members of her family should become sick and no physician near. Hydropathy ought to be taught in our schools, for the most valuable possession to anyone is his own body, and how many are able to take care of it? As the welfare and greatness of any nation depend on the health of its subjects, the Government ought to encourage the teaching of common natural hygiene thoroughly in the schools.

MASSAGE—ORTHOPEDY.

"Come forth into the light of things,
Let Nature be your teacher."—*Wordsworth.*

MASSAGE consists of manipulations of the body, either by hand, massage rollers or machinery. In all organic and nervous troubles the soft human hand is preferred to the machine for massage. But in obesity, certain conditions of stiff muscles, etc., machine massage gives good results.

The different movements are either strokes, clapping, hacking, kneading, vibrating, etc.

Self-Massage.—In some ailments you can massage yourself very effectually; for instance, with constipation, catarrh of the stomach,* torpid liver, sprained ankle (circular), headache (sideways), falling out of hair (backwards motion), neuritis (rub arm upwards).

No inflamed parts ought to be massaged.

Nervousness, a tender skin, babies in paralysis, around wounds and boils, and painful parts in rheumatism and gout, must be massaged with very gentle strokes, no clapping, hacking or vibrating to begin with.

The strokes of massage treatment should always

*See Figure 2.

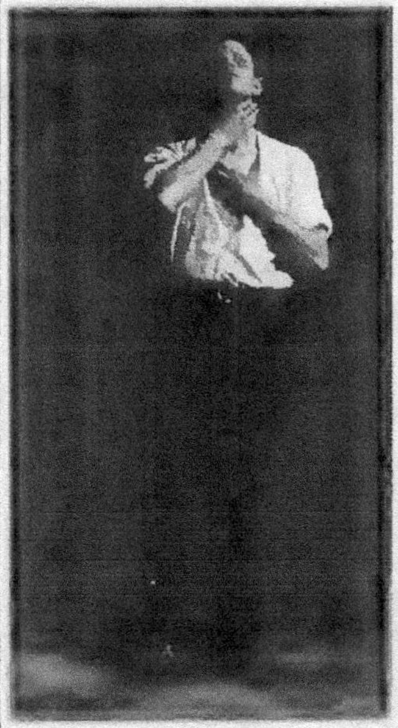

FIGURE 1. THROAT MASSAGE. 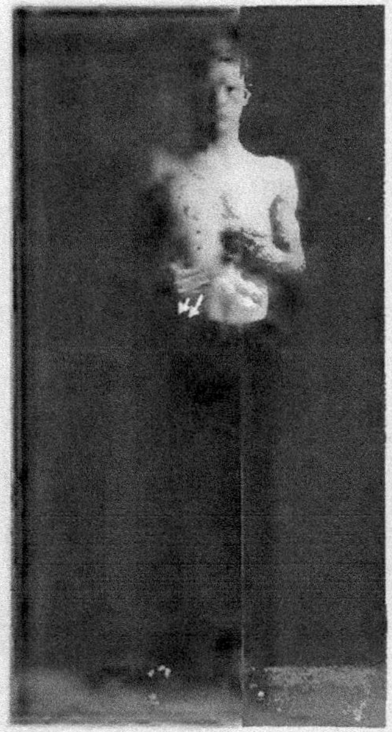 FIGURE 2. STOMACH MASSAGE. 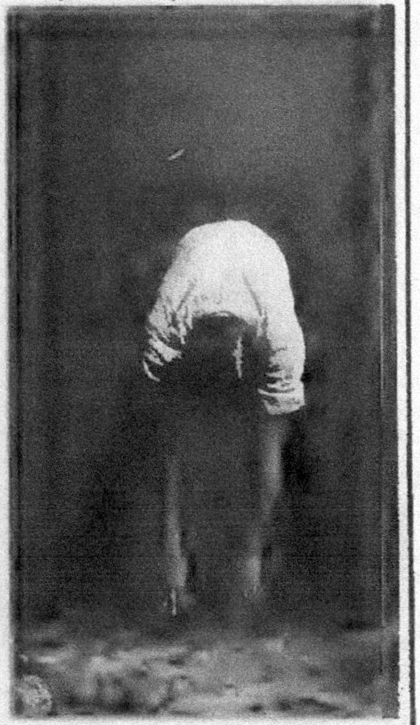 FIGURE 3. PULL THE BRANCH.

go towards the heart, namely, arms and legs upwards, back down, chest down.

Organic massage is best left to a scientifically trained *masseur* or *masseuse*. In cases where these cannot be procured, exercise bringing ailing parts into action help a great deal.

In all ailments where massage is forbidden, exercising ought to stop, too; for instance, in hemorrhages, fever, appendicitis, etc., until all danger is over.

Massage counts among the oldest forms of therapy, and even to-day we see savages practice it who scarcely commence to show the rudiments of culture.

Besides that, if we observe the animals, we see that they use it in rubbing bruises, contusions, etc. To show this I will relate here an experience in my life:

Several years ago I was visiting a friend, Mrs. A., in Texas. One day, as we walked up and down the spacious back yard, a large red ant ran toward me. I crushed it with my foot to and fro, so that it looked a flat, skinny piece, lying in the shade of the rear house. When I started on again I noticed another red ant coming to the crushed one, and going all around it, touching it with its head. I wondered when I saw the newcomer pulling it along, and said to my friend, "Wait, let us see; she will probably bury it." But no, she only pulled it out of the shade into the sun, and then began mouth and foot manipulations. I said to Mrs. A., "She probably embalms it with her saliva before burying it." After a few min-

utes another ant came, and she also began to push
her forefeet and mouth alternately against the sides
of the crushed body. So they both went on for about
twenty minutes, when the crushed ant's body grew
rounder and rounder, moved one leg after another,
and finally walked slowly away. I was greatly aston-
ished at the correct instinct of these little insects.
First the crushed body was dragged into the sun to
improve the impaired circulation and help the re-
expansion by its heat. Then they raised the crushed
body to normal roundness by incessantly massaging
the whole body. What a lesson from one of our
smaller insects!

Among the old cultured nations, Egyptians, Per-
sians, Chinese, Romans and Greeks, massage and
gymnastic exercises were highly cultivated.

The works of Oribasius, which were reproduced
with beautiful illustrations in Paris in 1851, are very
instructive, and show us that our modern Swedish
movements are a faithful imitation of Greek models.

Asklepiades was one of the most renowned physicians who highly cultivated the antique massage and
gymnastic exercises as healing factors. It was this
same Asklepiades whom we may regard as the father
of the physical dietetic therapy or Nature Cure, because he advocated all his life, beside massage,
water, light, exercise and diet as the main healing
factors.

In modern times it is the Central Institute for
Gymnastics, in Stockholm, founded by the gymnast
Ling, which is the source and nursery of modern
mechanotherapy.

Massage has also recently considerably developed, especially as "organic massage," in which the larger organs (lungs, liver, heart, uterus, etc.) as well as the smaller (eyes, ears, nose) are treated scientifically according to their anatomy, physiology and ailments.

The German and Swedish schools produce scientifically trained *masseuses* and *masseurs,* whose knowledge is founded on a thorough study of the anatomy and physiology of the human body.

Any physician who has drawn massage into his method of treatment soon finds that it deserves a prominent place in therapy, because very often pathological changes can be prevented and cured by it when they are but little or not at all influenced by other means. This is especially true in female trouble, where invariably an operation is advised, while we have in the Thure Brandt massage (internal), hydrotherapy and air-baths, the most effectual means for a thorough and agreeable cure.

Although the procuring of a scientifically trained *masseuse* or *masseur* is often more trouble than the writing of a prescription, a conscientious physician will not shun any trouble when he has found that many a chronic disease can be cured by massage when all other means fail.

How soothing it is to a nervous sufferer! How well he feels during and after its application! How strengthening to the weak before and after an operation! It makes the lame walk, the cripple normal, the complexion healthy, the bearing graceful, the lungs expand and grow healthy and strong. All the organs work normally by its help, and, thus strengthened, soon do satisfactory work independently. Combined with hydrotherapy, rheumatism and gout are cured thoroughly by it; so are swellings, varicose veins, dislocated and sprained joints, contusions, contractions, adhesions, curvature of spine, double joints, hemorrhoids, appendicitis, most female troubles, asthma, gall stones, kidney trouble, nervous diseases, etc.

In childbirth, massage is of the greatest help. It quickens the delivery, and in abnormal cases it brings about a normal position of the child, less suffering, no exhaustion, quick restoration of strength, prevention of blood flow and fever, besides the comfortable feeling it gives. All the most renowned gynecologists of Europe employ it, and there all midwives are trained to do it. Its use spreads rapidly, and we hail it with pleasure that most advanced physicians of all schools have incorporated it more and more into most of their courses of treatment.

Orthopedy, a branch of Nature Cure treatment, has been illustrated in our States sufficiently by Dr. Lorenz, two years ago, and we have saved many patients an operation by it. Thure Brandt massage is of the same order.

DIET.

Thorough mastication of your food brings roses to your cheeks and gold to your purse.—*Selected.*

Govern well thy appetite lest Sin surprise thee, and her black attendant Death.—*Milton.*

IT is really astonishing that in the twentieth century most people eat what they "like best," without considering that their health depends greatly on what and how they eat. If man had retained the original animal instinct, he would have his best guide in that. But as we have killed it by generations of wrong living, creating sickly, artificial appetites, we ought to endeavor to regain this natural instinct by a simpler, hygienic way of living.

Our blood is the natural food for all and each cell of our body, and as only a healthy organ can do good (normal) work, it is of the greatest importance that the blood, its food, be in a healthy condition. Our blood is formed from what we eat; therefore, our diet is not indifferent.

Liebig's albumen theory is at an end. The greatest scientists of our age prove that the most important part in our diet is the vegetable salts. Therefore, we ought to eat the same, and give our children from the first year of their lives sufficient of them. They are mostly contained in fruits and vegetables (especially lettuce and spinach). To make your baby strong give it, from the fourth month of its life, fruit juices, besides milk, and from its eighth month, vegetables (spinach especially, steamed and put through a meat grinder), besides milk and fruits, but no meat.

As there has been so very much written on this subject I will refrain from entering into details, and only say that our meals ought to consist mainly of fruits, vegetables, brown bread or whole wheat bread and nuts. Many people eat too much meat. Once a day is sufficient for anybody to eat it.

In diseases great attention should be paid to the character of the disease, and the diet prescribed accordingly, in order to effect a prompt cure. Meat creates heat, consequently it ought not to be given in feverish diseases.

The theory that meat gives strength is one of the causes of the degeneration of our present generation, as the greatest physicians (Lahmann, Boehm, Schweninger and others) have proved.

Most diseases of the digestive organs come from insufficient mastication of food. The haste and hurry of our times make people swallow their food very quickly, so that they may "get back to business quickly." In this regard the common mechanic is much better off, as he has at least an hour for his dinner, thus allowing sufficient time for masticating properly.

Recent researches and experiments of Mr. Horaz Fletscher have aroused the interest of the greatest physiologists and scientists of the world.

Mr. Fletscher, of Venice, is a wealthy man who studied dietetics from a mere philanthropic point of view. He tries to prove that a dietetic reform is the foundation of *all* reform, and that there will not be any "slums" after a reform in diet, clothing, dwelling, etc., has taken place. He says most people eat too much and masticate their food too little. If they masticated it four or five times as long, all stomach trouble would disappear, and with a better change of matter, naturally, almost all diseases.

Renowned men as Michael Foster (England), Professor H. F. Bowditch and Professor Chittenden (Yale) have tested his method, and Professor Chittenden gave recently his view of it in a very interesting article in the "Popular Science Monthly."

On account of the economical importance of this question the Military Department of the United States has ordered twenty men to spend their whole time and effort during several months by severely testing Fletscher's theory.

I myself have tried it with some of my patients with very gratifying results, and now impress it on all of them.

In kidney trouble, rheumatism, gout, anæmia, cancer, consumption, scrofula, skin diseases, etc., no meat ought to be eaten, but twenty or thirty nuts eaten daily as a substitute, until a complete cure is effected by the combined treatment of massage and hydrotherapy.

Eggs and old cheese produce much uric acid, except when with cheese is eaten either an apple or a potato, and with eggs some lettuce or other green vegetables.

Overfeeding and want of exercise are two of the main causes of disease. We ought to leave the table when we long to eat at least half as much more as we have eaten. Nearly everybody eats too many spices, especially salt and pepper, which make the blood impure and cause disease. Fruit and nuts, our most natural food, is eaten too little. Eat fruit at every meal, and if possible make one of your meals every day entirely out of fruit. Most people would improve their health by proper exercise and the following diet:

1. *Breakfast.*—Fruit, a cereal, wheat hearts, instantaneous tapioca or Force, etc., an egg, whole wheat bread, peanut butter, Lahmann's cocoa.

2. *Lunch.*—Various fruits, or one kind of fruit and a glass of sour milk (clabber), brown bread, cottage cheese, lettuce, radishes.

3. *Dinner.*—Fruit, steamed vegetables (especially often spinach and lettuce), rice, meat, dried fruits and nuts or a light pudding (fruits preferred).

One of the most easily digested and most nourishing foods is rice.

A great number of chronic diseases can be mainly cured by diet, especially diseases of the blood, of the digestive organs, and lung trouble.

Most people drink from habit, while they might learn from the animals to drink only when thirsty. A rabbit never drinks as long as it has fresh herbs to eat, for they contain enough water to supply the need of its body.

In nervous diseases, stomach trouble and hemorrhages nothing ought to be taken hot, but luke-warm.

Fast twice a month by eating only some fruits and nuts for a day.

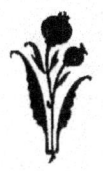

THE AIR-BATH.

Better to hunt in fields for health unbought,
Than fee the doctor for a nauseous draught.
The wise for cure on exercise depend;
God never made His work for man to mend.—*Dryden.*

THE air is our natural element, and in order to remain and grow well we ought to breathe pure air day and night. Not only should our lungs, but also our skin, breathe it. The skin is an organ whose work is to push impurities out of our bodies in the form of perspiration and poisonous gases, and in return to drink in the pure oxygen of the air through more than five millions of pores.

There are four ways by which Nature purifies our bodies from poisons—through the lungs, the kidneys, the skin and the bowels. But many people prevent the skin from acting by wearing too many and too closely woven garments; therefore, the lungs and kidneys must also do the work of the skin. They do it for a time without apparent harm, but the strongest organ cannot be overworked indefinitely and remain unharmed. A kidney or lung trouble is the consequence. In order to prevent this we should select loosely woven clothes, and every morning and evening we should give our skin a chance of free action by taking an air-bath in our room.

Undress as much as possible and open all the windows. According to the temperature, keep more or less in motion or rest. In hot weather much motion is not necessary, while in cool and cold weather it is imperative. For this purpose we would advise an exerciser put up at the post of your door, and suggest that your physician prescribe the necessary exercises and their duration. These air-baths will prove beneficial both to the healthy and the sick. The motion prevents chilliness and helps better circulation of the blood. Every person needs these baths more or less, and millions of people would be well instead of sick if they would take them regularly, beginning with two minutes, increasing to at least half an hour, every morning and evening. They are the main element in the cure of anæmia, obesity, weak lungs, skin diseases, scrofulous and nervous diseases. In the Nature Cure Sanitariums of Germany they have regularly built air-baths in the open air, which are favorite places of all the patients. Very feeble invalids and nervous patients, who can scarcely bear the mildest form of water bathing, can stand two air-baths during a day, and are greatly benefited by them.

These baths are the safest and most agreeable way of hardening ourselves; persons who take them regularly scarcely ever take cold. Consider all the savage nations, who on an average are healthier than any civilized nation. Can you imagine them doing without their air-baths? No, not even the inhabitants of the colder zones. In Dr. H. Lahmann's booklet about ''The Air-Bath'' there is a very interesting illustrated account about the air-baths of the heathen Esquimaux on the east coast of Greenland.

He says: "The observations made by Frithjoff Nansen on his expedition to Greenland amongst a people living in a state of nature may assist us. Nansen noticed that the heathen Esquimaux on the east coast of Greenland undressed in the evenings in their skin tents, and so unconsciously took regular air-baths, although the tents were but poorly warmed by cod-liver oil lamps. Nansen rightly observes that this instinctive air-bathing while in tents was a necessary compensation for the harm done by the impermeable fur clothing.

"This opinion of Nansen's has been shown to be correct by the condition of the Esquimaux on the west coast of Greenland, who for some time now have been under Danish rule and influenced by Christian missionaries. The latter naturally teach their followers that this air-bathing in tents, occupied by several families in common, is indecent and wrong, while in other cases, owing to the adoption of many of the European vices, the people have become so poor that they can no longer build skin tents, but are compelled to live in caverns. The result of these changes is an increased mortality, principally owing to lung trouble, and Nansen believes that the whole of the Esquimaux population on the west coast will in a short time be destroyed. Let us take a lesson, therefore, from the Esquimaux!"

THE SUN-BATH.

"The sun is all about the world we see,
The breath and strength of every spring."—*Swinburne.*

NOTHING in the universe can live and thrive without the sun. The health, growth and color of all plants and animals depend upon it, and thus it can be easily understood why the sun has been worshiped as a god.

Among the various kinds of healing methods it is especially the fast-spreading Nature Cure, in which the sun, in the form of light and sun-baths, is so effectively used. Although the old Greeks and Romans took sun-baths in their "Solariums," it is only within the last twenty-five years that the latter have been incorporated in a systematic, scientific way into medical treatment, with more and more surprising results of its great healing virtues. In all Nature Cure Sanitariums of Europe, especially in Germany, special sun-baths are built.

The effect of the rays of the sun on our bodies varies according to their application. If they reach our skin through glass, we receive only the beneficial heat and light; but if they reach us through open space directly, they cause also a powerful chemical change of matter in our body. As in all chronic diseases the change of matter in our body is insufficient, these baths are one of the most valuable means in curing chronic diseases.

The sun-bath proper is taken in the following way: In the open air, surrounded by a 10 to 12-foot high close fence or wall; on an elevated platform mattresses are laid in long rows. On these the patients expose their bodies to the sun, either bare or wrapped in a light blanket. The head is protected by a bench or umbrella, etc. The air must be calm and the thermometer up to at least 95° F. in the sun. As this is the most powerful of all treatments, on account of the great chemical changes taking place in the patient's body, these baths must be given with good judgment as to the individual case. There must be a cold compress upon the forehead. People with a tender skin ought to be covered with cheese cloth or a light blanket.

Imagine your body to be square, and let the sun shine on each of its sides for ten minutes. In very weak patients only five minutes for the first time. Then rise and wash the body off with cold water, and rest for at least half an hour; weak persons rest two or three hours.

Sun-baths are used especially for rheumatism, gout, neuralgia, lung trouble, diabetes, dropsical swellings, flybetus, rickets, anæmia, scrofulousness, lupus and various other skin diseases. Even in recent years physicians had no idea of the effect the sun had on the human body. As to its revolutionary power in stirring up dead poisonous matter, burning it up and excreting it by perspiration, a sun-bath is even more powerful than a Turkish or Russian bath. He who has never taken a sun-bath may feel a little reluctant "to bathe in the sun," but after once having felt its delightful sensations he certainly regrets that he cannot take it oftener. On an average, a whole sun-bath ought only to be taken every twelfth or fourteenth day. But when only a part of the body takes it as lungs, legs or arms, it may be taken more frequently; but as its effect depends mostly on the constitution, a physician ought to be consulted for minute directions. Many people might think it strange to be advised to expose themselves to the rays of the sun in summer, when everybody longs for the shade. But the difference is in being undressed. Why do the animals often seek the sun for their resting place in summer? How different are the faces of people who are almost always out of doors, under the influence of sun and light, from those pale, sickly looking beings who are like prisoners, nearly always locked up in their houses. A room into which no sun shines is not by far as healthy as one into which it comes. Put a plant into the cellar, and it loses its color and strength. Put it into sun and light again, and it regains both. Fruits cannot ripen without the sun, and man requires it equally with the plants.

It is to be regretted that in many countries they can be taken only in summer. But let us be benefited by them whenever we can, for pestilence walks in darkness and dirt. Sunlight is death to disease germs.

PHYSICAL CULTURE.

Motion is Life,
Inactivity is Death.

A S all organic life depends on the normal change of matter, it is of the greatest importance to retain it in health and to regain it in sickness, and this is done by physical culture. To have the proper effect, observe the following rules:

1. Remove all tight and heavy clothing.

2. Take only those exercises which suit you individually. Let your physician prescribe them for you.

3. The exercises must be done quietly, without haste, but with force of the muscles. If you are weak, do it as well as you can. Every day you will be able to do them better.

4. Never overdo, but stop when tired. It is well to begin with a few motions and increase them as best you can.

5. If the exercises cause *lasting* pains in your muscles, it is a sign that you overdid, and you have to make a pause; then begin again with *very gentle* movements.

6. The best time is always one-quarter or one-half hour before a meal and two hours before you retire.

7. During the pauses, put your hands on the hips and breathe deep and long.

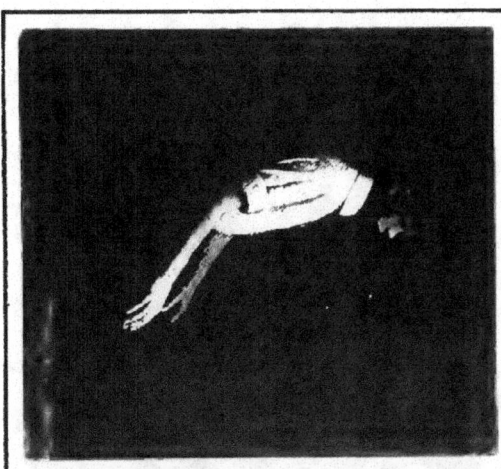

FIGURE 4. SIT ON HEELS.

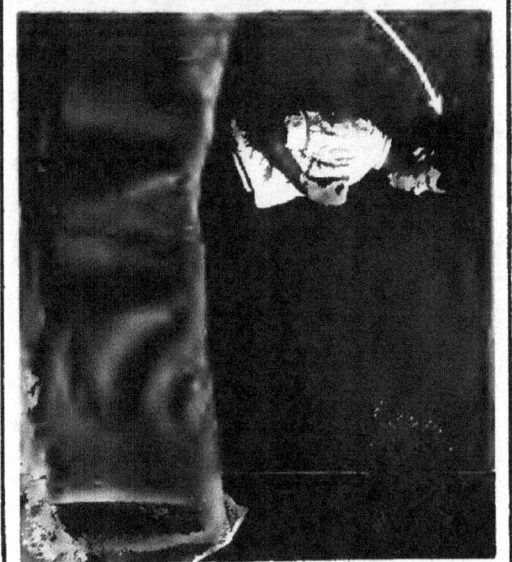

FIGURE 5. SITTING UP.

8. If breath and pulse go very fast, stop a little while until calm.

9. Number and length of time for exercises have to be prescribed by your physician.

10. If you do not understand anything about physical culture and its effects, do not undertake it during a serious illness without instruction from an experienced person. To perform a complete cure, hydrotherapy, massage and proper diet have in most cases to accompany it.

11. Patients who are sick in bed can do them also in a lying or sitting position, or with the help of another person.

12. Besides many other benefits, physical culture improves the sleep and the appetite, increases cheerfulness and gives new joy in life.

Pull the Branch.[*]—Stand with feet apart, raise arms straight above your head, breathe deep (imagine you have to pull a branch down in front of you), and bring down hands to touch the floor, if possible, holding your breath, and your knees stiff. Count five, erect yourself again, and let out your breath.

Good for all imperfect abdominal functions, constipation especially, and it strengthens the nerves and muscles of the back.

Sit on Heels.[†]—Stand with heels together, raise heels, bend knees, stretch knees, let heels sink.

[*]See Figure 3.
[†]See Figure 4.

This exercise is especially helpful in stiffness, lameness, rheumatism, gout, etc., of legs, and prevents stiffness of old age.

Waist Turn.—Stand with heels together, legs stiff up to the hips. Turn upper body *slowly* around to the right as far as possible, count five, and go around slowly to the left; count five there, then return to right, etc., twenty times each side, if strong. Weak patients may begin with three or four times each way.

This exercise is made more effective when performed on a piano stool, upper body held stiff, and lower part moving right and left. It is especially effectual in liver trouble, hip disease, vertigo (go very slowly) and constipation.

Sitting Up.*—Lie flat on your back and raise yourself into a sitting position without the help of the arms. If it is impossible, put, at the beginning, a pillow or some other weight on feet, or put feet underneath a piece of furniture, and by degrees this will become unnecessary.

This exercise is very helpful in all stomach and abdominal disturbances and functional weaknesses.

Pick Up Pebbles.—Bend down with stiff knees to pick up something, walk three to five steps and put it down again; walk a few steps and repeat till tired.

This exercise is especially good, and should be used very extensively with piles, constipation and all nervous abdominal affections.

*See Figure 5.

Water Treading.—Let two inches of cold water run into your bath tub; step into it and tread down the water in a walking step, raising each time the sole of the foot above the surface of the water. Do this every morning and evening, first day one minute, increasing one minute every day up to five minutes. Then continue all the while with five minutes. When you stop, dry the feet. If they feel warm, everything is all right. If not, exercise or rub them till warm. In a short time they will be warm directly after the water treading. You must not let them stay cold. If necessary, take a hot foot-bath to make them warm. Very nervous people begin with tepid or cool water, and go gradually to the cold.

Water treading is a very effectual means against cold feet, heart trouble, chilblains and frozen feet.

Head Turning.*—Close your eyes and turn your head around to the right *very slowly* in as complete a circle as possible. Then for a time around to the left. If it causes dizziness you did it too quickly.

Very useful for stiff neck, congestion of blood in the head and headache from this cause, nervous dizziness, fat neck, throat trouble and "old woman's lump."

Leaning Leg Exercise.†—Stand three or four feet away from the foot of your bed; lean hands on it. Then let some one take hold of your ankle and raise your leg into a horizontal line, without your resistance. Then draw down your leg with stiff knee and the other person withholding in a measure, according to strength of patient. In the beginning the assistant ought to withhold but little.

This exercise strengthens most muscles of the body and has a strong "drawing off" effect on the abdominal organs.

A. Knee Separation.

B. Knee Joining.

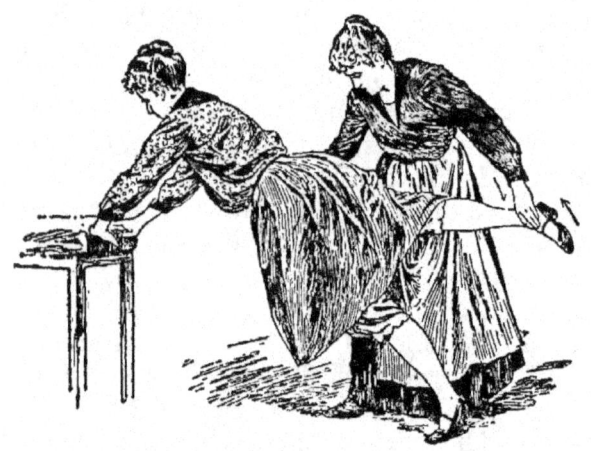

(Figure 7.)   Leaning Leg Exercise.

A. Resisting Knee Movement.—As picture shows, the patient lies on her back with raised knees. The physician or assistant at her side separates her knees, while she resists and raises her pelvis until the hips are pretty straight and the weight of her body rests only on feet and upper back. Then she puts her knees slowly together again, while the assistant resists.

This exercise is repeated three or four times.

B. The position is the same as in A, with the only difference that the assistant holds her hands outside of the knees, pressing gently while the patient separates them, raising herself as in A. Then the assistant gently pushes them together again, while patient resists.

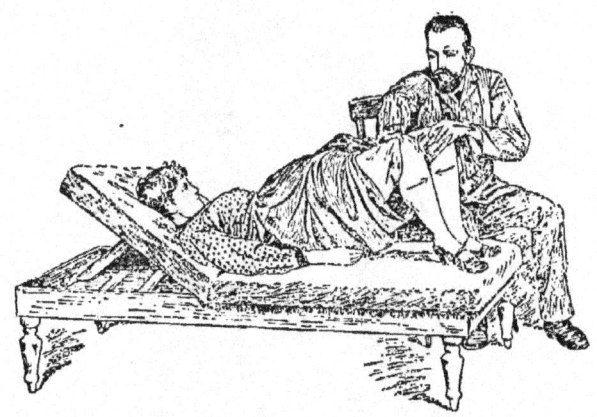

(Figure 8.)   Resisting Knee Movement.

This is done three or four times.

These exercises shorten all the muscles of the small pelvis, so that bowels, bladder, etc., can do better work. They are used directly after having replaced the prolapsed uterus (womb), vagina and rectum; also by a retroversion of the womb. Both applied at the same time draw off the blood from the abdomen.

Knee Bent Hand Pressing.—(R e s i s t i n g Movement.)　One foot rests with its upper side on a chair,
back of patient, on which also the assistant stands.
The patient's knees are the same distance from the
chair; she stretches her arms straight upwards and

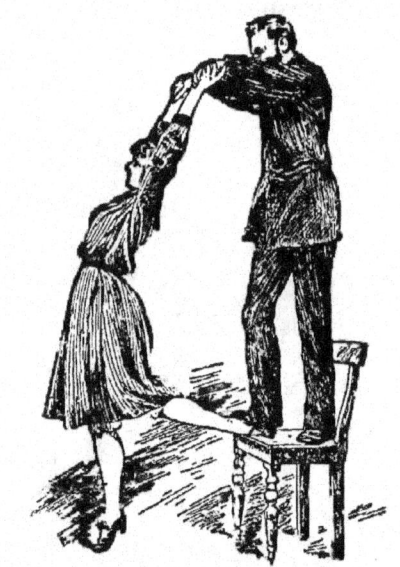

(Figure 9.)　Knee Bent Hand Pressing.

backwards, bending spine.　The assistant puts his
thenars (lower fleshy part of the thumb) upon cor-
responding thenars of the patient, and his four
fingers around the side of her hand.　She holds his
hand likewise.

Now the patient raises herself on her toes, then

slowly bends the knee, while the assistant presses (or helps) her gently down, and the rest of her body remains in the same position. Then she raises herself again (he resisting a little), and then lets heels down to starting position.

This is done alternately three or four times with each leg.

In order to have the wished-for effect, it is of the greatest importance that during the whole exercise the pelvis is put forward, that the assistant does not press too hard, and that the patient does not bend her arms.

This exercise draws the blood powerfully to the pelvis and to the legs, and is used with much success in amenorrhœa (absence of menstruation). It must be used only when advised by a physician, because there are cases when the menstruation would weaken the patient (anæmia, etc.).

CHEERFULNESS.

It is a known fact that the mind controls the body to a great extent. This is especially so with nervous people, and in our time most people are more or less nervous.

We all know that worry and fear are the greatest poisons for the body; so is cheerfulness one of its best medicines. To this many people will answer, "That is easier said than done, and how can you be cheerful when you are sick or unfortunate?" But I tell you, you can if you *want* to; for "where there is a will there is a way.'' This is *my* proverb, and I have practiced it since my youth, when my dear mother taught it to me. It helped me to total recovery when I was a nervous wreck myself. I have had many nervous patients who were helped materially to their restoration by it. So, for instance, even in the dreadful hysterical epilepsy, most of my patients had an attack by indulging in sad and worrying thoughts. After I told them to recall several especially joyful or funny events in their lives, and when sad thoughts would assail them to discard them at once for the former, they have, in most cases, been able to avert an attack. We all should practice this until it becomes a habit, and we are cheerful all the time.

Hand in hand with it, naturally, a hygienic way of living should go, for an improving physique influences our mind favorably too.

Last year I treated a young lady for kidney trouble. She was always in an unpleasant mood, discontented, grunting, complaining, frowning and pouting. After I had treated her for some time her relatives and friends complimented her and me on the total change in her disposition. She was like another being, always cheerful, polite, bright, contented and full of fun. Recently her aunt said to me: ''Doctor, I must compliment you for having so totally changed my niece. It is a very remarkable cure. Last year I was glad to see the change, but feared it would not be lasting; but as it has lasted for a year, I hope it will continue. It makes us all very much happier to see her so cheerful.''

So let us all do, improve our health and grow and remain cheerful. Thus we shall be much more lovable sisters, brothers, wives, husbands, mothers and fathers, enjoy ourselves much more, make others happier, and create a comfortable, peaceful, enjoyable tone in all our homes and wherever we go.

GENERAL HYGIENIC RULES.

1. Practice deep breathing all the time.

2. Take an air-bath every morning and evening.

3. Sleep with open windows throughout the year.

4. Take two leisure walks every day, but if you follow a sedentary life take as much exercise out of doors as possible in the mornings and evenings, and also some exercises in physical culture.

5. Neither smoke nor chew tobacco.

6. Drink no coffee, tea, nor alcoholic drinks.

7. Masticate your food well; twenty times each soft bite, and thirty, each hard bite of food.

8. Do not eat much meat, but live chiefly on fruits, vegetables and nuts.

9. Do not ride a bicycle; it weakens the heart.

10. Do not wear heavy underwear, nor sleep under heavy bed clothes.

11. If possible sleep alone, as it is unwholesome to sleep with another person.

12. Do not worry! It is the worst poison in the world.

13. Look always on the bright side of life, and cultivate cheerfulness in thought, society and books.

If you follow these rules you will grow healthier, stronger and happier every day.

DIRECTIONS FOR SUCCESSFUL NURSING.

1. Make patient comfortable; undress him and put him on a clean bed with a hard mattress.

2. Keep the windows of the sick room open day and night, except during the time the patient is exposed in bathing, etc. In cold weather the room ought to be heated 65° to 70° F.

3. Let the surroundings of the patient be as quiet as possible.

4. Never waken the patient for treatment, even if the fever be high.

5. Be gentle, cheerful and thoughtful of all the needs of the patient.

6. Have the patient's bowels moved at least once every day, by a small lukewarm enema, in a *lying* position, held from five to fifteen minutes, followed after the moving of the bowels by a small remaining enema.* In typhoid fever, appendicitis, strictures, peritonitis, inflammation of the female organs, etc., from three to six enemas should be given daily, with remaining enemas following every evacuation.

7. Do not put much covering on a feverish patient, except when he has chills, as he is already too hot from fever. A feverish patient cannot take cold.

8. Never give a patient alcoholic drinks, except by special prescription of the physician.

9. If anybody is wounded or poisoned, and no doctor at hand, look up chapter on "Wounds and Poisoning," to give the first aid.

*See Figure 10, and refer to "Remaining Enema."

10. If you or any of your dear ones should feel sick, and you do not want to send for the doctor at once, apply a trunk pack and calf pack for the night, or for at least three hours during the day, preceded by an enema, and followed by a cold sponge bath, or a warm tub bath, 90° F. Thus you can in most cases prevent sickness, and in no case can it ever do harm. Repeat if needed.

11. If a patient's head be hot and his feet cold, put a hot water bag or a heated brick to his feet and cold compresses to his forehead—the latter renewed every three minutes. Do not use an ice bag, as it causes a paralytic state of the blood-vessels, and thus does more harm than good.

12. The most strengthening, the most easily digested food, and that which contains the most nourishment in the smallest form and gives least work to the digestive organs is almond milk. (See chapter on "Hygienic Cooking.") It is used in all hospitals and sick rooms in Europe when the patient cannot take anything else, needs nourishment but must spare the digestive organs, and where he has to be fed through the rectum in the form of an enema.

13. In long cases of sickness, where the patient must not be moved much, to prevent bed sores keep a basin of cold water underneath the bed where he is lying, renewing it every morning and evening. If possible, wash his back frequently with cool water.

14. To avoid much moving of a very sick patient, have his nightgown open the whole length of the back, so that it can be put on like an apron, pushing it under his sides without moving him.

15. Wear yourself light cotton clothes. They are more cheerful for the patient, and do not gather the germs of disease like woolen clothes.

16. When with a patient, do not sit on his bed— that might oppress him—but on a chair, where he can see you without turning his head.

17. Do not talk too much, nor busy yourself continually about the room—both make the patient nervous.

18. For all WATER TREATMENT, as baths, packs, etc., note the following rules:

(a) The colder the water the shorter its applications should be.

(b) The patient's body should be warm when any cool or cold water treatment is given.

(c) The room in which the treatment is given should be warm.

(d) All packs and hot baths should be followed by a cold or cool sponge bath, or a warm (90° F.) tub bath.

(e) Never take a bath directly after a meal—wait at least an hour.

(f) Do not give any water treatment directly after great excitement, fright, anger, etc.

(g) If a child *shuns* a cold water treatment, make it easy for him by beginning with a warmer temperature than the prescribed one, and gradually make it cooler. If it is only from *naughtiness* that he resists, then insist upon his taking it.

PARENTAGE.

The most important, the most honorable task which can be set any woman is to be a good and wise mother.—*President Roosevelt.*

Children are idols of hearts and of households,
They are angels of God in disguise.—*Milton.*

TO be a mother is the greatest, the noblest state of woman. It is much to be regretted that comparatively few know and treasure its importance, and that so many avoid motherhood. Most of our greatest men—writers, artists, statesmen—as Milton, Goethe, Washington, Napoleon, Richard Wagner and many others, attribute their success to the beneficial influence of the noble character of their mothers and wives. There can be no greatness, no financial or scientific success in a nation without healthy, noble mothers to give it healthy children; for only in a healthy body lives a healthy soul, and only a healthy mind can achieve greatness in any walk of life. Therefore every mother ought to do all in her power to produce healthy, noble offspring. The physical health is given the child by the mother's hygienic way of living during pregnancy, and by the child's being reared in a hygienic way. This I shall explain further on.

The mental strength and qualities of the heart are imparted to it by the mother's practicing them dur-

ing pregnancy, the father before that time, as well.
If you want your child to be musical, hear and practice good music as much as possible during pregnancy, putting your whole soul into it. The same
with mathematics, economy, diligence, oratory, etc.
To have a good-natured, lovely child, practice char-
ity, love, forbearance, patience; think kindly of
everybody; never let your temper overcome you.
Abstain from all bad habits, alcoholic drinks, smoking, etc., and think with love of the coming baby.
If you do this, you will without doubt have a child
of fine character and great talents. To give it a
healthy body be guided by what I shall say concerning pregnancy.

Prenatal influence is one of the greatest powers
in the reproduction of our race, and therefore of
vital importance. As to a great degree you can
model your children by it, do it in the way to produce
a healthy physique and a noble character in them.

The greatest misery I have seen during those long
years of my practice came from immorality, which
is the greatest curse of *civilized* nations, for most
savage nations are not immoral. Here I remember
an event from my own life.

When I was a young girl there came to our zoölogi-
cal garden for a number of years a Mr. Bergmann,
with about 20 or 30 savages, every summer another
type. They were there for show on a large lawn
inclosed by a low fence, living as they did at home,
hundreds of people looking on.

One day I went there with a friend, but at the

first sight of those almost nude savages I felt
shocked and as if I had to run away. But then I
thought that that would make me too conspicuous
and I might be laughed at. My friend seemed to feel
the same and said: "Oh, how shocking to have all
those almost naked people before children and everybody."

We stayed and watched one of their meals, their
work, etc.

When we left I said to my friend: "I have learned
something to-day. I think those savages are better
than civilized people, for I am convinced they are
not immoral." I watched them all the time, and none
of the men, not even the youngest, cast as much as a
licentious look towards those almost nude girls. And
I, being always modest in dress and behavior, had
often to experience vile looks from our "civilized"
young men, even clerks in stores, etc. I wonder if
that is a *"blessing"* of civilization? During my
study and long years of practice I have become convinced that our children are born with a tendency to
immorality. Proof: little babies practicing self-
abuse. And this is caused by frequent intercourse
during pregnancy. Most savages regard this as a
crime, and spare their wives during that time. If
they did not refrain they would produce children
with abnormal sexual tendencies, just as civilized
parents do.

PREGNANCY.

First of all, discard your corsets, and wear instead
a well-fitting muslin waist—not too tight, and with-

out steel in the front. Have buttons on the waist, to which you can attach your skirts. Attach the stocking supporters on the sides, above the hips—not in front, for there should be no pressure on the abdomen.

As soon as you know you are pregnant, stop frequent marital relations, as intercourse in this state produces in the child a tendency to nervousness, as well as licentiousness. Why, the wild animals do not indulge during that time, and is man to be less humane than an animal?

THE LAUDABLE ENDEAVOR OF VARIOUS SOCIETIES TO DECREASE THE GREAT EVILS THAT ARE THREATENING THE TOTAL RUINATION OF FUTURE GENERATIONS BY THE RESULTS OF IMMORALITY AND OTHER VICES, WILL NEVER EFFECT ANY RADICAL CHANGE SO LONG AS THEY ATTACK THE BLOSSOMS AND BRANCHES OF THE TREE AND LEAVE THE ROOT UNTOUCHED. THE ROOT MUST BE KILLED BY TEACHING THE YOUNG HOW TO PRODUCE AND EDUCATE A NEW GENERATION, FREE FROM LICENTIOUS AND OTHER IMMORAL TENDENCIES.

WHY DO SAVAGE NATIONS NOT NEED HOUSES OF ILL-FAME NOR INSANE ASYLUMS? BECAUSE THIS LICENTIOUS TREE, WITH ITS POISONOUS VICES, DOES NOT GROW AMONG THEM, AND THEY DO NOT HAVE A DRUG STORE AT EVERY CORNER. FOR AILMENTS THEY TAKE A TEA OF HERBS, JUST AS WHOLESOME AS OUR VEGETABLE SOUPS, BUT NO MINERAL, METAL MEDICINES WHICH CONTAIN STRONG POISONS, AND THEREFORE THEY ARE HEALTHIER THAN WE.

*   *   *   *   *

Be as modest in married life as you were before its consummation; it will insure you the lasting love of your consort.

Let all your time for pleasure be spent in out-of-door sport; leisure walks, picnics, sleighing, coasting, skating, etc.

Practice deep breathing all the time, especially after each meal.

Live out-of-doors as much as you can.

Sleep with open windows throughout the year.

Do not ride a bicycle. Do not reach high, nor lift heavy things without holding your breath.

Do not regard yourself as a sick person, and do not lie around if well; but exercise as much as possible, especially in the open air.

Eat very little or no meat; if none, as a substitute eat 20 nuts every day, masticating them well; or eat some peas or beans.

Eat sparingly of things containing much lime, as salted fish, salted meat, milk, etc. The lime makes the bones of the baby hard and childbirth painful. To produce a *small* head in the child, and consequently an *easy* birth, live mainly on fruits, nuts, vegetables and cottage cheese. Drink as little fluid as possible, for too much water in the womb will cause it to expand unduly and consequently lose its contracting power—so important in childbirth—and make you so large that you shun going out.

Do not eat sweets or many fried dishes.

Brown bread is better than white bread.

Do not season your food highly.

Mingle in cheerful, intelligent society, and indulge in good literature.

Take frequent air-baths.

If your circulation be poor, practice water treading. (Page 55.)

If constipated, eat whole wheat bread and practice exercises as directed under "PHYSICAL CULTURE."*

Take during the first half of your pregnancy a sitz bath, 90° F.—fifteen minutes, four times a week; in the latter half, take one every day. Once a week, during the whole time, take a warm 95° F. tub bath, for ten minutes—then reduce the temperature until you can stand it without discomfort. Never take any bath shortly after a meal.

If your breasts are not normally developed they should be treated by massage to increase their glands. If the nipples are not normal, they ought to be made so, even before pregnancy, by massage, breast glasses, etc., so that you will be able to nurse your child. It is very much to be regretted that so few mothers are nursing their own offspring, as there is nothing that can replace the mother's milk. This is why so many babies die in the first year of their lives. From generation to generation it will grow worse, because a young mother who has not been nursed by her own mother has degenerated breasts, and so will be less able to nurse her child than her mother was. If the father of a young wife was given to drink she will in most cases not be able to nurse her child. Healthy normal breasts are one of the greatest charms of female beauty, but if the

*See Figures 4, 6, 15.

present conditions continue there will be nothing but artificial busts in a not far distant future.

If you follow these directions, you will have an almost painless childbirth, and be rewarded with a strong, healthy child.

CHILDBIRTH.

Childbirth ought to be painless, for it is not a disease; and it can be made almost so by a hygienic and an appropriate living during pregnancy. Statistics show that 98 per cent. of all births are normal, and a normal birth should, as with animals, be painless, or cause no more discomfort than an evacuation of the bowels. Why then is it not painless among the people of civilized nations?

1. Because our women are weakened by a wrong way of living, by a want of outdoor exercise, by their style of dress (corset), etc.

2. Because the child's head is too large for the passage. This fact has been proven by Dr. Lahmann. What makes it too large? The mother's incorrect way of living creates in the child before birth a fatty degeneration, obesity and too large a head. You should not be proud of a fat, heavy child. Compare the newborn calf of the prairie with the average newborn child. The first is nothing but skin and bone, the baby is a lump of fat. The calf and the thin baby increase in weight from the beginning; the fat baby decreases from the beginning during several weeks. Another proof of No. 1 is seen in savage nations.

For instance, a savage tribe is on a wandering trip. A pregnant woman feels her time has come. With some of the other women she goes behind a bush, where she soon, painlessly, gives birth to the child. She then washes it in the nearest brook or spring, ties it on her back and continues her trip. Why is childbirth so easy with her? Because she never wore a corset, and every day had plenty of outdoor exercise.

Nature Cure wants all women to come back to this original strength, for then mothers will look forward to childbirth with pleasure, instead of with fear and trembling. Therefore away with the corset! Arouse yourselves to daily out-of-door exercise, combined with deep breathing, ball playing, rowing, skating, coasting, sweeping or shoveling snow and mowing. If you have no time for these, walk to the market, to your place of business, etc., instead of riding, and practice deep breathing all the way. Why is consumption not raging in Japan as in other countries? Because every Japanese child is taught deep breathing systematically, and practices it all his life, is always in the fresh air and eats very little meat, but an abundance of rice, fruit and vegetables.

For the birth of the child, choose the sunniest and most airy room in the house. Let there be two beds in this room, so that the mother can rest alternately upon a fresh bed.

Everything must be very clean, and the windows open day and night, not only because fresh air will help to keep the mother well, but it will also give the baby a good supply of oxygen in its lungs with its first breath, as a health-giving foundation for healthy lungs. Before birth the baby breathes through its liver. The omission of these precautions is one of the causes of so rapid an increase of consumption in our day.

When you think your time has come, and you feel warm, take a cleansing bath of 90° F. and an enema, for the bladder and the rectum ought to be kept empty during childbirth.

No internal examination should take place except in very urgent cases of an unexpected obstacle to childbirth, because it is often the cause of puerperal fever, and even death of the mother.

After the birth, both mother and child need a very thorough cleansing. The baby must be washed first in two separate basins, in warm water, one for its eyes and one for its body. The greatest care must be taken not to let any particle of the impurities which cling to the child's body enter its eyes, as they cause inflammation of the eyes and often total blindness. After it is washed quite clean, pour a pitcher of cool or cold water over its body; wipe it and put a navel band and clothes on it. Its daily bath after this should be at 90° F., followed by a cooler pour on the upper part of its back. This greatly strengthens the nervous system.

The mother is lifted into a sitz bath of 90° F., and after ten minutes lifted out again, put on a fresh bed, and a strip of absorbent cotton, 3 x 8 inches long, dipped in clean water, put between her legs and the lips of the pubes, from the anus to the pubic bone, and covered well with dry, clean flannel. Renew this compress every four or six hours; it is a means of preventing puerperal fever. It causes the fresh arterial blood to flow profusely towards these parts, to cleanse and heal the sores of childbirth. Besides this it absorbs the cleansings and other impurities, thus preventing their entering the blood. A sitz bath after childbirth is worth gold for its refreshing, cleansing, strengthening and soothing qualities. After this the mother generally falls into a sound, refreshing sleep. She should have such a sitz bath every day for two weeks after childbirth; after that, every second day for six weeks.

If the mother be healthy, she can be up the second day for a short time to exercise a little about her bedroom. Then from day to day a little more, avoiding overexertion.

As to her diet, she ought not to eat any animal food during the first weeks after childbirth, but may eat, if well, during the first days, milk toast, soups of cereals, spinach soup, fruit juices, almond milk, etc., and later on add green vegetables, bread sticks and nuts.

Every mother ought to nurse her baby. It is beneficial to the mother in many ways, and it is due to the child. There is no complete substitute for it as a nourishment for the child. It is, to a certain degree, a guarantee of health and strength.

With our weakened nervous generation it very often happens that in childbirth labor is insufficient to give birth to the child. It may enter the small pelvis, but there it stops. The mother's hands, feet and nose are cold, her pulse grows weak. She fails more and more, and the application of instruments seems necessary. As it is the want of warmth in the body which is the cause of impeded labor, our effort must be to give it warmth. For this purpose we lift the mother into a sitz bath of 100° to 105° F. We put her feet in a foot-tub full of water, 108° to 110° F. On the abdomen protruding out of the water we put large hot compresses. Over the upper part of the body we spread a blanket, and over her knees hot dry flannels. Besides these, we let the mother drink hot sugar water, very sweet. Soon, more color comes in her face, and a stronger beating of her pulse shows returning warmth. Labor sets in again, and in most cases with desired effect.

Length of sitz bath depends on the amount of labor, and the progress of the birth. Half an hour in most cases is sufficient. During this time the high temperature of the water must be kept up. Heat, thus applied, not only makes childbirth quick, and saves total exhaustion and an *instrumental* birth to the mother, but it also softens all those lower active parts, vagina, perineum, so much that their rupture is prevented. The position the mother keeps in the sitz bath is better than any other, and the child naturally comes to its destined opening by its weight and the law of gravity. All physicians should try the hot sitz bath, and they will not regret it. In houses where there is not a sitz bath, a deep wash-tub, put close to the wall, may be used.

Birthmark.—If your child has a birthmark of a purplish red color, as you sometimes see in people's faces, lick it frequently from the very first day of birth, and by the ninth day it will have permanently disappeared.

HEALTHY CHILDREN.

The childhood shows the man,
As morning shows the day.—*Milton.*

WE are all the product of our surroundings. Therefore let everything that influences our bodies and minds be pure and healthful. Be a healthy mother by leading a hygienic life, and nurse your baby. If you cannot nurse your baby, feed it with cow's milk, to which you add either the juice of fresh fruits or berries, or a little water and milk sugar. With a soft rag, wrapped around your first finger, wash out its mouth after every meal.

When the child is four months old, give it twice every day some fruit juice, besides nursing it. At eight months, decrease the times of nursing still more, and give it, in addition to milk and fruit, some green steamed vegetables, especially spinach, carrots, oyster plant, asparagus tips, etc., all steamed without spices, and put through a meat grinder and feed with a spoon. By degrees, increase this fruit and vegetable diet; in the ninth month, add some cereals once a day, and wean the child during the tenth month.

Keep the child clean by bathing it all over daily, and washing its private parts after every action of the bowels.

Almost all savage nations regard it as a crime to

have marital connection while the mother is nursing the child. They can control themselves better than the men of civilized nations do, I am sorry to say; and these savages are humane towards their wives and children. Even the wild animals refrain then, and why should man be worse than the animals of the forest and the prairie? Poor wife, who either has to have a baby every year, or become a nervous wreck by using harmful preventives!

Let the child's food for six or eight years consist chiefly of fruits, steamed vegetables and nuts, with a few cereals. No meats, no sweets!

Until it is three years old give it a daily tepid bath, 90° F., followed by a cold or cool pour. After that, give it a bath every second day. The private parts should still be washed after every movement of the bowels and bladder.

During the child's first months of life, notice how often it wets its diaper, then train it in this way: Take it up before the time comes and hold it over a chamber, making sh, sh, sh, sh sounds until it urinates. If you do that regularly the child will soon imitate you by trying to make the same sound when it feels it must urinate. Thus not only much diaper washing is saved, but the child will have strong, healthy abdominal organs.

Never induce the baby to walk. Let it crawl as much as possible, and when it feels able to walk it will raise itself at a chair, bench, baluster, etc., and walk without your assistance. If you make it walk before the little legs have strength to carry the body the child will be either bow-legged or knock-kneed. Although they can be cured, I think prevention is better than a cure.

So many mothers rock, swing, or jolt the baby when it cries, and infer from its ceasing to cry that this motion did it good, but it only stopped because the mother *stunned its brain* with her violent shaking. Do you think that does it good? Do not accustom the baby to be carried, but put it in a baby buggy out-of-doors all day long, pinning its cover to the sides of the buggy and to its jacket with safety pins. Do not excite it in any way, and do not let strangers shake and kiss it.

Dress the baby in this way: A little chemise of cotton or linen—no flannels—a thin cotton underskirt with bodice, and over this a slip of wash goods, wide at the neck. In hot countries, and here in summer, a slip is sufficient. Put yourself in its place, and think what suffering much clothing causes you in summer. In cold weather, when you take it out— and it should be taken out every day, in any kind of weather—put a loosely woven jacket or sacque around it. At home you always create a summer heat; therefore beware of overdressing the baby. Do not let it wear either shoes or stockings in the house, and when out of doors only sandals. If you regard the remarks of others about not wearing stockings, let them be as thin as possible, and of a very loose weave, so that the skin can act properly. The child will always have warmer and healthier feet than those children whose feet are incased in shoes, stockings and leggings, and consequently are pale, damp, cold and bad-smelling. *Your* child will not have these discomforts nor a poor circulation. The experiment is worth your trial.

Exercise the baby's muscles and lungs in playful gymnastics. Later on by out-of-door exercises, especially ball games, sleighing, coasting, skating, running, swimming, rowing, etc.

When the child enters school, ask the teacher to give it a seat near an open window. Wherever there is a crowd there is a bad, poisonous air, and I am very sorry to say that most of our schools are insufficiently ventilated. In most of the schools in Germany the recitations continue for fifty minutes. After each lesson all of the pupils are required to go into the yard, and run for ten minutes. One pupil in each class has to open all the windows of the class room, regularly, before leaving it, and to close them when the pupils return. This is an excellent sanitary arrangemnt and prevents much sickness, especially consumption.

Let your child sleep with open, screened windows all the year round. In summer the screens keep out the flies, and in winter the snow and the rain.

Do not take your child to the theatre, or to balls, etc. Watch its literature so that it does not read anything which will cause nervous excitement, as the "Arabian Nights," and books of a similar character, which give the child wrong ideas of things, and by portraying impossible happenings keep its brain in a whirl of excitement. The reading of such books often causes dreadful nightmare, and even attacks of epilepsy. Give it wholesome modern literature. Love stories are also injurious. They create a sexual lust, which too often leads to self-abuse and all its ruinous subsequent effects.

Let no child of yours ever smoke, or drink any alcoholic beverage.

Teach it early to do things for itself, even if you keep a house full of servants. Such a course helps to form a strong, independent character. Teach it to be strictly obedient; a contrary course makes children physical and moral weaklings.

Further, teach your children natural hygiene in a comprehensible way. Do not think they are too young for it. They should also be properly taught in the schools. It is frequently presented in such a way that no good results from it. It is simply a book knowledge of anatomy and physiology that is poured into the child, instead of a *practical* hygiene, that even a child of three years could be made to understand by object lessons, which it will remember and practice all its life, after the habit has been formed.

As the best teaching is done by example—stirring up the monkey habit in us—be a model to your children in everything you desire them to acquire.

SICKNESS.

Sickness is a disturbance of the normal functions of our bodies, caused in most cases by impurities (poisons) either from without our own body (in-

6

fection, etc.) or created in it. Therefore the main thing for a cure is to drive out the poison. This is done best in acute, feverish diseases by trunk and by calf packs, and in chronic diseases by making the patient sweat either through a vapor bath, dry pack, or a bed steam bath.

Very nervous patients and those with an organic heart or lung trouble should not take the cabinet vapor bath, but the bed steam bath, to be followed by either a cool sponge bath or a tub bath, 90° F.

So in case any of your dear ones feels sick, and you do not know what is the matter, feel his body and see whether he is feverish. Ask him whether he has any pain, whether his bowels have been moved that day, and whether he has any appetite. If there be pain anywhere put an extra wet cloth on it, in the pack. If his bowels have not been moved, give him first an enema, after that, treatment as directed above.

If his head be hot, put a cold compress (wet cloth) on it, and renew it every three minutes.

If he be feverish do not feed him, but give him cool drinks frequently; almond milk, fruit juices, etc.

Keep the windows of his bedroom open day and night. Thus treated in time you can very often prevent a long, serious disease.

If after one treatment the patient feels better, but not well, repeat it the following day. Do not give him anything to eat until he is really hungry.

In *no* case can you do any harm with the above treatment, but you may greatly benefit the patient.

PART II.

DISEASES TREATED

ALBUMINURIA.

Albuminuria is a kidney trouble. There are different kinds. If it accompanies an acute disease, look for the treatment of that disease; otherwise the treatment is as follows. A hygienic way of living, a mild vegetarian diet, milk, almond milk, moderate eating, tepid or warm and air baths; much out-of-door exercise will at least improve, if not entirely cure it. Kidney massage is also helpful.

ANÆMIA.

Anæmia is poor blood to a high degree. If the case is not a very bad one, it is sufficient if the patient passes most of her time in the open air, exercising moderately, and taking air baths. Her diet must consist of fresh fruits, green steamed vegetables, especially spinach, lettuce, radishes, turnip-greens, brown bread, or bread sticks, etc. Drink milk, buttermilk, almond milk, fruit juices.

To prevent constipation, take an enema every day *at the same time,* in a lying position—a pint of water, 70° F.

In pernicious anæmia the patient ought to be moved to the country. There she should lie out-of-doors all day long; to be wheeled about sometimes is also helpful. The want of exercise is substituted by general massage, until the patient is strong enough to exercise sufficiently. If the stomach and bowels are affected give the patient a stomach pack of 74° F. every second night. Should this disturb her sleep, or if it does not grow warm, discontinue it.

An anæmic girl should not marry until thoroughly restored.

ANGINA PECTORIS (Nervous heart pain).

First of all regulate your diet to avoid attacks of pain. Smoking and drinking of alcoholic drinks, must be avoided; also coffee and tea. Highly seasoned food should not be eaten. Let the diet consist of green steamed vegetables and fruit. If kidney trouble or rheumatic affections be the cause, meat should not be eaten. For the evening meal eat but little and nothing that is very hot.

A general massage, combined with a scientifically applied heart massage, vapor baths, gentle exercises, water treading and the avoiding of all excitement, worry, anger, fright, etc., will gradually cure the disease if no incurable organic trouble is the cause. At time of attack, give the patient hot foot, hand and heart applications.

The patient should avoid all violent exercise, heavy lifting, running, etc., but have every morning and evening resisting motions with arms and legs, and if he cannot have a *masseur,* massage his heart himself, rubbing from the breast bone towards the left arm.

APPENDICITIS.

Appendicitis is an inflammation of the appendix, accompanied by much pain. The swollen appendix can be felt in the right lower side of the abdomen. Its most frequent cause is constipation. It is generally accompanied by fever, quick, hard, small pulse, and restless sleep. In the beginning, give the patient every hour an enema of 80° F. until profuse evacuations follow; these to be followed, each by a remaining enema of 65° F. Do not give any purgatives, as they irritate the inflamed intestine still more. Further, give the patient abdominal packs day and night, first renewed every half hour; later every two hours. They reduce the inflammation, prevent an extended peritonitis and suppuration of the connective tissue back of the appendix, besides soothing the pain and decreasing the fever. Sitz baths of 90° F. have the same effect, and may be taken three or four times a day.

The patient should have only a mild fluid diet— milk, buttermilk, almond milk, fruit juices, brown soup No. 1, and apple sauce. If the case is accompanied by much vomiting, feed the patient during the first days with small remaining enemas of almond milk. This treatment is always satisfactory.

After the fever is gone a gentle abdominal massage is applied.

APPETITE (Lost).

A loss of appetite generally occurs with acute diseases, and with an acute catarrh of the stomach. It also results from overeating, and from unwholesome, poisonous foods.

First of all, give the stomach a rest by refraining from all food, and remove the cause.

APPETITE (Abnormal).

With some diseases there comes an abnormal appetite, a "ravenous hunger" shortly after a bountiful meal. The main cure for this condition is to eat very little and frequently in the beginning, and by and by a small meal at the regular time, applying stomach and calf packs, at least during the night, and if possible during the day. Massage of the digestive organs quickens the recovery. Add air baths and plenty of outdoor exercise.

Old cases of hysteric epilepsy have been cured by us in this way.

ASTHMA.

Asthma is difficult breathing. When an attack comes, remove from the patient all tight clothing, and especially all pressure on his chest. Open all the windows in his room, and on a quiet day the door also, to cause a gentle circulation of the air, which is agreeable to the patient. Then sprinkle much water on his face and chest, and rub his whole body with dripping wet towels.

If the attack comes during the night, let the patient put his feet in a basin of cold water. If the attack is a long one, heat water quickly and put vapor compresses on his chest and back, renewing every ten minutes. If you have a vapor cabinet, give the patient a vapor bath directly, instead of the vapor compresses. It is of great help to many patients to press their thorax (chest) together during the attack.

If the patient is able to do some exercises let him follow those which are termed stick exercises,* or give him chest exercises which are done in this way: the patient sits on a stool; you put your foot behind him on the stool, and your knee against his back. Seize his wrists and draw his arms forward and upward, backwards and downwards, while the patient breathes deeply, resists a little the pulling up of arms going up, and exhales and pulls your resisting hands going back and down.

To cure asthma thoroughly the patient should go to a Nature Cure sanitarium, where the causes of the disease can be systematically treated.

BASEDOW'S DISEASE (Morbus Basedowii).

This is a nervous disease with quickened heart action, swollen thyroid glands, and goggle eyes.

The patient needs general and local treatment, the former consisting of cool sponge baths, and baths of 90° F., alternate days, a mild diet, regular move-

*See Figures 11 to 14.

ments of the bowels, warm feet, living much out-of-doors, air baths, sun baths, bodily and mental rest, and a daily nerve massage, and of the thyroid glands.

To cure the goggle eyes promptly, put an eye pack on the eyes every night, and take eye baths six to eight times during the day, preceded by massage of the upper eyelid, done in the following manner: Seize the upper eyelid between two fingers and make the motion of a coffee mill with it. These eye treatments also prevent more serious eye trouble.

BOW-LEGGED CHILDREN.

As prevention is better than cure, do not allow your baby to stand or walk much before its little legs are strong enough to carry its body. But when its legs are already bent put to their outer side a thin, narrow strip of wood covered with some soft material, and tie it at both ends with soft bands of ribbon. The pieces of wood must not cover or rub the ankle bone, nor the knee. Tighten the bands a little every day. Along with this, give him two or three times a day a gentle leg massage, rubbing legs upwards, and keep him in the open air playing in the sand all day long, if possible, but do not let him use his legs much. Give him healthy food, proper clothing, etc., and he will grow strong.

BROKEN BONES.

Remove all clothing from broken parts. Then place the patient so that the broken arm, leg, or whatever it may be, has a pillow or sand sack, etc., underneath it, the surface of which you can adapt to the normal form of the broken part, that it may rest upon this pillow.

If the bone is not entirely broken and no displacement took place, it is sufficient to put some splints to the injured part, attached with strips of wet linen. Over these wrap dry flannel and keep the patient on a firm but not soft bed. This is especially necessary with broken ribs, because the success in the healing of the bones depends, to a great extent, upon the first adjustment of the broken parts of the bones.

If a bone is entirely broken, let a second person hold the normally lying end, while you put the other part of the bone back to its place. Then tie around the place of fracture, three or four times, a wet bandage of three or four inches in width, but not too tightly on account of the swelling. Over this, tie two or three suitable splints. Over this, wrap again three or four layers of wet bandages, then dry absorbent cotton, and a dry flannel bandage. Cover the patient and let the injured part have complete rest.

Whenever the heat of the injured parts makes the patient restless, remove flannel, cotton and upper wet bandage. Then wet the first bandage a little with a sponge, and put over the splints again a fresh wet one, and replace the cotton and flannel bandage.

After three or four days, all the bandages are removed, the injured parts bathed with warm water, and bandaged again as in the beginning.

In complicated fractures the injured parts are massaged before bandaging them, in order to remove and bring to absorption the blood which has accumulated there and make possible a perfect adjustment of the bone.

After the bones have knit, remove all bandages and massage and exercise the injured parts regularly, in order to prevent their stiffening.

If accompanied by fever, look up "FEVER."

BURNS.

Should your hair or clothes catch fire roll burning parts up quickly and tightly in a rug, a blanket, etc., to extinguish the flames, then put burnt parts directly into tepid water; later on, into cold water until all pain has gone, which sometimes takes only a short time; in serious cases, hours. This is the only sure and quick cure for burns.

Parts which you cannot hold in water, the face for instance, ought to have water continually poured over them until the pain has ceased. If tepid water is not at hand, begin directly with cold. Holding the burnt part in flour soothes the pain. Blisters from burns disappear while holding them in the water. If you have large blisters in a place which cannot be held in water, lance them and keep a wet rag around them for a long time, renewing it frequently.

Cover *open* wounds either with a soft rag dipped in sweet oil or tepid water; keep it on until granulation

takes place. Then dampen it well, remove it carefully, and cover the wound with soft, cold, wet linen,
which you must frequently renew.

Burns treated in this way heal more quickly than
by any other method.

CARBUNCLE AND FURUNCLE.

The carbuncle is a very large boil. Its cause is
impure blood. Our main aim must be to eradicate
the poisons from the system. For this purpose we
give the patient daily, for a time, a bed steam bath
or a vapor-bath on a chair, followed by a bath
of 90° F. for eight minutes, with a pour on the carbuncle. Day and night the carbuncle must be well
covered with a pack three times its size, in order to
influence the surrounding parts. This pack must be
renewed when it becomes painful. The wet part
may be from six to ten layers in thickness. If possible, let the patient lie on the side where the carbuncle is, as in that position the pus flows out better.

After the boil has opened, press it gently in order
to thoroughly remove the impurities; wash it frequently with warm water.

Keep the room well ventilated, and give the patient
a very mild diet as indicated under "FEVER."

CATARRH OF THE STOMACH (Acute).

The symptoms of catarrh of the stomach are loss
of appetite, thirst, belching, vomiting, dry coated
tongue, headache, weakness and sometimes fever.

In *slight* cases, eat very little for a few days, or nothing at all. Drink every half hour a little cool water. Take moderate out-of-door exercise on warm, sunny days. Three times a day and during the night an abdominal pack and foot packs, which remain two hours in the daytime and all night if comfortable. Give stomach massage twice a day, five to eight minutes.*

In more serious cases, accompanied by fever, treat the patient as follows:

From 8 to 10 A. M., abdominal and calf packs,† followed by a cool sponge bath.

From 10 A. M. to 10.30 A. M., rest.

10.30 A. M., a trunk bath, 90° F., fifteen minutes.

From 11 A. M. to 1 P. M., abdominal and calf packs.

1 P. M., an enema of 72° F., and after the evacuation, a remaining enema.

From 1.30 P. M. to 3 P. M., above-named packs.

From 3 to 3.30 P. M., rest.

3.30 P. M., bath as above.

From 4 P. M. to 5 P. M., rest.

From 5 P. M. to 7 P. M., packs as above.

From 7 P. M. to 7.30 P. M., rest.

7.30 P. M., enemas as above.

8.30 P. M., packs as above, which stay on until morning unless the patient grows restless in them, in which case they are renewed.

*See Figure 2.

†See Figures 17 and 18.

During the feverish period, give the patient only a fluid diet, consisting of almond milk, fruit juices, Quaker oats soup, milk, buttermilk, Dr. Lahmann's pure cocoa, etc.

Massage of the digestive organs after the fever is over will help to restore their normal functions.

You can apply self-massage by kneading the abdomen, with fine results, if done for eight minutes every morning and evening, in a lying or standing position.

CATARRH OF THE STOMACH (Chronic).

Chronic catarrh of the stomach generally develops from the acute, and its symptoms are the same, but not so pronounced.

1. Eat often, but little at a time; chew the food well.

2. Avoid highly seasoned food of every kind.

3. Avoid old cheese, potatoes, gravy, fried foods, pie, meats, coffee, tea and alcoholic drinks.

4. Do not drink anything at your meals, nor half an hour before eating; nor for two hours afterward.

5. Eat frequently instantaneous tapioca, rice, oatmeal, wheathearts, corn, barley, peas, beans and other *green* vegetables which do not cause any discomfort, stewed fruit, apple sauce, soft boiled eggs and toast.

6. Eat no meat except a small portion of a tender fowl or game.

7. Drink once a day a cup of almond milk.

An hour before your noon meal put on the stomach and calf packs, and keep them on until an hour after the meal. Put same packs on at night.

Morning and evening take a trunk bath of 90° F., an hour long; hotter water for the feet.

Stomach massage is of great importance, if it can be had; it quickens the complete recovery. One kind of massage the patient can do himself to great advantage is shown in picture.*

CATARRH OF THE BOWELS.

Catarrh of the bowels is caused by wrong diet, cold, emotions, or by the spreading of an inflammation near the bowels. Its main symptom is diarrhœa; further, pain in the abdomen, flatulence and sometimes loss of appetite accompany it.

It is treated the same as catarrh of the stomach, except that abdominal packs are applied and abdominal massage given, besides two enemas, and six remaining enemas daily till normal and free evacuations follow without any mucus.

CATARRHAL PNEUMONIA.

This disease is treated the same as bronchial catarrh.

CHOLERA INFANTUM.

This disease is chiefly caused by wrong diet. Its symptoms are diarrhœa, loss of appetite, vomiting, pain in the abdomen, with the child growing pale, thin, dim-eyed and looking much older.

*See Figure 2.

This disease, so fatal to babies, becomes less so when the mother nurses her own child and keeps it clean. If she·cannot nurse it, it is best to feed it with cow's milk to which is added one-sixth part of fresh fruit juice, or one-eighth of water and milk sugar. I have seen very good results from feeding babies on almond milk mixed with equal parts of water in which figs were boiled.

During cholera infantum it is sometimes advisable not to urge any food upon the baby, but to give it an enema followed by frequent small (one to two teaspoonfuls) remaining enemas of almond milk. In very obstinate cases of diarrhœa it is advisable to cleanse the bowels frequently by enemas (one to two cups), followed after evacuation by small (one spoon) remaining enemas. Hot compresses on the abdomen and baths of 95° F. help greatly to hasten the recovery.

When all danger is over give the child daily one or two baths of 90° F., or 85° F., for strengthening, and often brown soup, Quaker oats soup, mushroom soup, etc.

COLD IN THE HEAD.

Take either a sun-bath, vapor-bath, dry pack, or sweat, followed by a warm 90° F. bath.

Take much out-of-door exercise and keep your body in an equal warmth. If you are not hungry, fast a few days, and drink only fruit juices and almond milk.

Take two enemas daily, if constipated.

During the night put packs on throat, stomach, and calves of legs.

COLIC.

Go to bed to get all parts of your body into an equal warmth.

Take a remaining enema five or six times through the day.

Rub your abdomen around the navel like a coffee mill, gently at first; later on, deeper. Put hot compressses on your abdomen and eat a little of a mild diet, rice, stewed fruit, etc., or fast. If the pains are very great, take a hot bath (108° to 112° F.) or a vapor-bath. In most cases vapor compresses are sufficient.

CONSTIPATION.

Take every morning, *exactly at the same time,* an enema. If not very successful in the beginning, take two or three a day, each evacuation being followed by a remaining enema.

More important than the above is the abdominal massage, which alone is able to restore strength to weak bowels, and to substitute the abdominal pressure. If you cannot have a well trained *masseur* or *masseuse* for it, do it yourself, kneading and rubbing the abdomen for ten minutes, mornings and evenings. Use also physical culture exercises,* and

*See Figures 3, 4, 5.

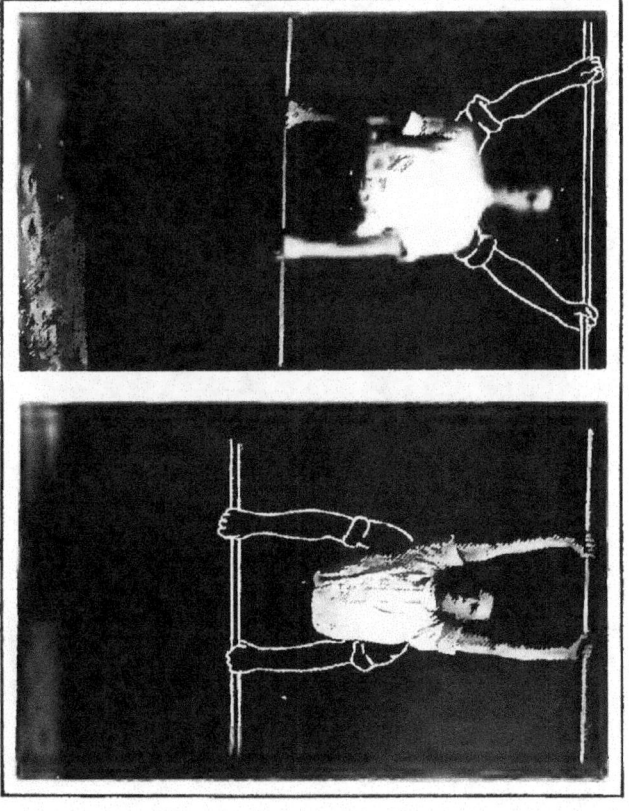

FIGURES 11 and 12. STICK EXERCISES

"pick up pebbles," page 54, every morning and evening till tired.

Swimming and rowing are of great benefit. Chew your food till it is a fluid.

Eat freely of fruits and nuts, dates, figs, honey, whole wheat bread, bread sticks, and vegetables as peas, beans in purée form. Also the fruit soups as given in the chapter on "Hygienic Cooking."

Garden work is excellent if the patient can have it.

CONSUMPTION (Lungs).

Consumption is only infectious by the sputum (expectoration). A tendency in this direction can be inherited, or it can be acquired as an outcome of a chronic inflammation of the lungs (pneumonia). Generally the patient coughs, expectorates, has a quickened pulse and breathing, night sweats, fever, and often pain in the chest.

Not only Nature Cure physicians, but those of the allopathic school, have come to recognize that it is not medicine that cures consumption, but fresh air all the time, air-baths, and a diet of fruits, green vegetables, nuts, cream, milk, eggs and butter.

No disease is easier prevented than consumption. As it is spreading so rapidly, the Government should establish rules and regulations which would cause its decrease. In one of these, Germany might be followed. There, in all the schools, after each lesson of fifty minutes, ten minutes is given for recreation—a run in the yard. At the same time all the windows in the class rooms are opened wide. In rainy weather a trot in line under long colonnades would accomplish the same results.

Further, the law ought to forbid consumptives to marry, as their children may inherit the tendency for it. These two regulations alone would greatly lessen the number of cases. If regulations for the proper ventilation of factories were enforced, the disease would be well-nigh extinguished.

Advanced consumption is incurable.

In the first stages it is cured by the following: Every morning and evening take an air-bath as long as possible, at least half an hour.

Out-of-door exercise with long, deep breathing in *pure* air, all day long.

No heavy, tight, closely-woven underwear, but a light, open mesh fabric, or a chemise, or shirt alone, in summer time. No furs, and an overcoat only in very cold weather.

A meatless diet, as stated above.

Massage and packs of the lungs (see Figures 22 and 23), or any affected part, will considerably quicken the recovery.

With consumption of the throat, spare your voice, gargle frequently, or take mouth baths of lemon juice and water.

Throat and calf packs during the night.

A warm 90° F. bath once a day, with a throat, chest and back pour, 40° to 80° F., ought to be taken, too.

Whoever does the above faithfully will recover thoroughly, and grow strong and healthy.

CORNS.

Take a hot foot-bath (100° to 106° F.) of soap water, thirty minutes; wash the feet with cold water and remove the softened corn with your penknife or finger nail. If it does not come off entirely, take another foot-bath to soften the rest.

Instead of the foot-bath you may put thick, wet packs for several nights on the corn to soften it; remove in the morning as much of it as is soft. In two or three mornings the corn will have been removed.

COUGH.

A cough is a symptom of a disease, not a disease itself. Look for this, and treat it as directed.

CROUP (Membranaceous).

Membranaceous croup is an inflammation and swelling of the mucous membrane of the throat, with an excretion covering it which is coughed out as soon as the effect of Nature Cure treatment has changed the dry, hard cough into a loose one.

It generally begins with the symptoms of a slight catarrh, then, as a rule, follow sudden attacks of a hard cough, with difficult breathing, approaching suffocation, accompanied by a peculiar, penetrating, long sound.

At first these attacks come at long intervals, then they are of more frequent occurrence. When the blood becomes overloaded with carbonic acid, the breathing grows shorter and shorter, and not so loud.

The patient appears better, but on the contrary, this is the most critical time, and death often follows in an apparently quiet slumber.

Croup is treated in the same way as a bronchial catarrh, only we give the bath 90° F. three times a day, morning, noon and night, and have the patient gargle with cool water every half hour.

If a severe attack comes on in the night, put the patient directly into a bath of 90° F., cooled down to 85° after a few minutes; then a cold pour on the patient's body, chest, back and throat. The water in the bath must reach a little above the navel of the patient. Even in the height of an attack, do not hesitate to give this bath, for then it is most needed, and has saved many a life.

Continue the treatment for some time, even after all the symptoms of croup have disappeared.

CURVATURE OF SPINE.

Fresh air day and night.

Every day a cold sponge bath, or a tub bath of 90° F., with a back pour of 60° F.

The diet must consist mainly of fruits, vegetables and nuts; no meat.

Twice a day massage the back downwards and pack the back and calves during the night. Further, apply spinal bandages and a stretching apparatus. Use exercises called "stick exercises."*

*See Figures 11 to 14.

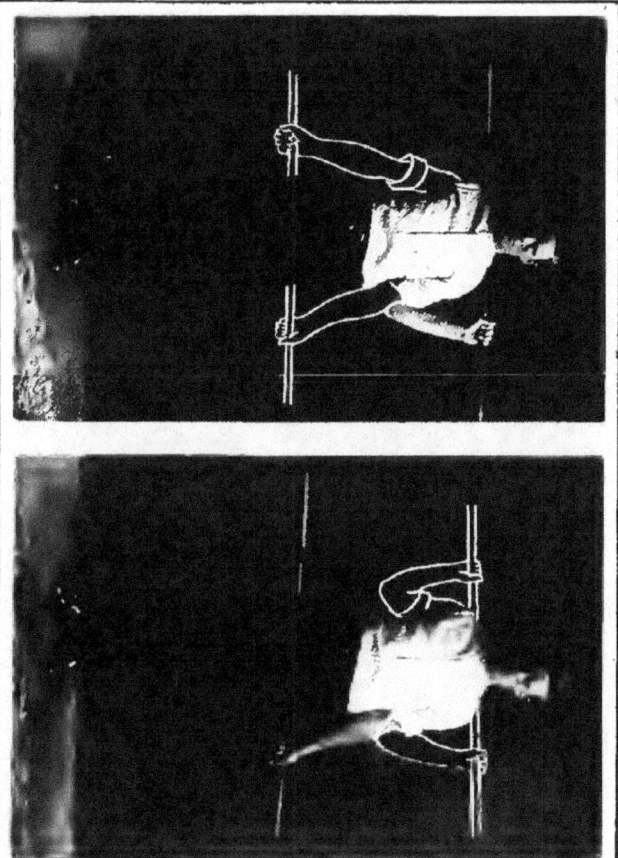

FIGURES 13 and 14. STICK EXERCISES.

DANDRUFF.

In slight cases, dandruff disappears through the following treatment. Draw a straight line from front to back of head, near the ear. Wrap a soft rag around your forefinger, dip it into the yolk of an egg, and rub it well into the scalp at the drawn line. Then make lines successively, one inch apart, all over the scalp, rubbing the egg well in. Then take a clean rag and warm water and rub along each line with it. Finally wash the whole scalp and hair twice in warm water and ivory soap. Then rinse it well with warm water, and dry it. If two or three of these treatments do not remove the dandruff, it is deeper rooted, and a series of vapor-baths, a fruit and vegetable diet, and general massage must be applied.

DIABETES MELLITUS.

This peculiar disease comes from insufficient action of many organs, with much sugar in the blood and urine.

Its causes are various—infectious diseases, a cold, high living, wrong diet, insufficient mastication, or an organic hurt may bring it about. Sugar in the urine is its main symptom. Indigestion, constipation, vertigo, headache, and loss of appetite generally accompany it.

The diet is here of the greatest importance. Do not eat much at a time. Take morning, noon and night a tumblerful of well whipped bonnyclabber.

Along with this, drink almond milk and fruit juices.
Eat moderately fruits and green, steamed or raw
vegetables, as lettuce, celery, tomatoes, radishes, also
eggs, chestnuts, nuts, potatoes in a limited quantity,
but not much starchy food; no meat, no sweet things
of any kind, no coffee, tea, nor alcoholic drinks.
Besides this we must make the skin act. Give the
patient every morning a cold sponge bath, followed
by gentle rubbing in wiping him. Then give him,
according to his strength, either every day, or every
other day, a full tub bath of 93° F. for eight or
twelve minutes. These baths help the change of
matter and prevent the disagreeable itching and car-
buncles.

Strong patients may take a sweat every twelve or
fourteen days, or a vapor-bath.   .

Take regularly sun- and air-baths; they burn up
the sugar in the system and greatly improve the
blood.

One of the greatest healing factors in diabetes
mellitus is a general, scientifically applied massage.
If you have no one to give it, rub arms and legs of
patient gently upwards, back and chest downwards,
stomach as shown in the illustration,* and the abdomen around navel; his left side down and his right
side up, each part for five minutes.

If patient is strong enough, he may do some physical culture exercises, according to his strength.†

Patient ought to eat little and masticate it long.

*See Figure 2.
†See Figures 3, 4, 11 to 16.

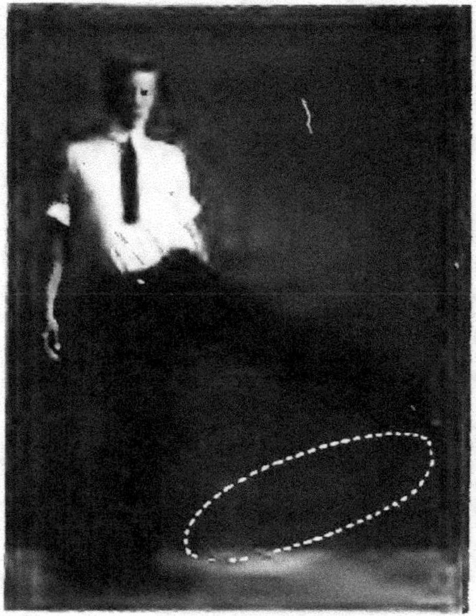

FIGURE 15   LEG EXERCISE

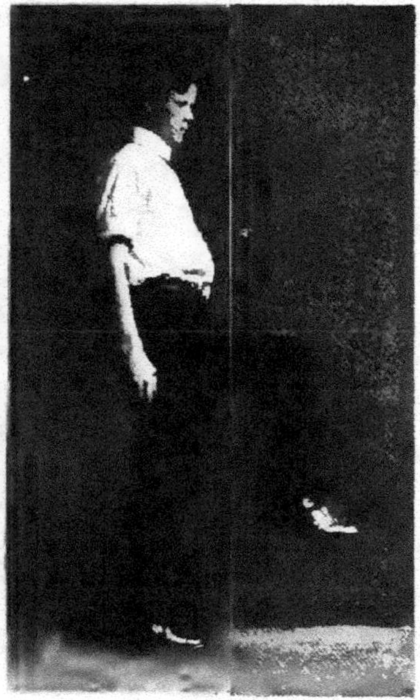

FIGURE 16   KNEE EXERCISE

Medicine can do no good to the patient, but a stay in the mountains, and still better in a Nature Cure sanatorium, is of great benefit.

Certain symptoms of ·this disease, as carbuncle, furuncle and constipation, need special treatment. Look them up under each named heading.

DIARRHŒA, FLUX, DYSENTERY.

All three are treated much alike.

If a diarrhœa is not accompanied by alarming symptoms, it suffices to put the patient on a diet of instantaneous tapioca soup, barley soup, almond milk, brown soup No. 1, milk toast, etc., besides applying enemas 80° F., with remaining enemas following the evacuation.

For flux and dysentery, give the same diet; add cooked huckleberries, either fresh or dried, and blackberry wine. Instead of the water enemas, give them of thin oatmeal soup from three to six a day. If an evacuation occur, let it be followed by a remaining enema.

Besides these, give the patient several sitz baths a day, 90° F., for ten or fifteen minutes. They soothe the pain, decrease the inflammation, regulate the movements of the bowels, and make the circulation normal.

In case the patient is very weak and sensitive, even towards tepid water, it is better to choose mounting sitz baths; that is, make them of a temperature of 92° F., adding hot water until it is 105° F., twenty minutes long.

If you have not a sitz bath, put from four to six vapor compresses on his abdomen, each ten minutes duration, equal to forty to sixty minutes duration. These latter serve to remove severe abdominal pains and to help in removing poisonous food which may have entered the bowels.

Cramp-like pains at the anus are relieved by local vapor compresses.

A scientifically applied abdominal massage helps greatly to cure the disease.

DIPHTHERIA.

Diphtheria is an acute disease caused by a poisoning of the whole organism, with special characteristic symptoms of the mucous membrane of the upper breathing channels, also of the intestines. The disease may originate of itself, or it can be caused by contagion.

Many authors regard diphtheria as a purely local disease, where the poison is received first by the mouth only, and much later entering the blood. We think differently, and believe that the poison first enters the blood through the breathing organs, or through the digestive organs, and later forms those local symptoms mentioned above.

This theory is proved by the circumstance that diphtheria has generally a period of incubation, in the form of a feverish, general sick feeling at a time when there are not yet any anatomical changes noticeable in the throat.

Treatment.—We can only prevent contagion by avoiding direct contact with the breath of the patient, and by continual good ventilation in the sick room. In accordance with our theory of the cause, we try to do the following:

1. To prevent or stop the formation and absorption of products of decomposition in the blood.

2. To bring out of the body in the shortest, quickest and least dangerous way those products of decomposition already present.

3. To increase the power of resistance of the organic albumen to decomposition.

4. To decrease quickly the local processes of inflammation and decay, and the consequent poisoning of the blood.

Number one we reach especially easy from the beginning period of incubation, by giving every day three or four enemas of half a pint of water of 72° F. After every evacuation, we give a little remaining enema in the form of a few spoonfuls of colder water, 63° F.

Number two is accomplished by making the skin act. The skin is decidedly a much larger and more dangerous field of disease than the minor organs, or even the small throat. Nature herself points to the pores of the skin as a way for excreting the products of decomposition, and our practice has taught us that these cases generally improve quickly, and end well, where from the beginning there was good and frequent perspiration. To this end we apply trunk packs,* renewed every two hours, and packs of the legs,† renewed every four hours, followed each time by a sponge bath or wash off, of those parts which were packed with water, of 70° F.

If the patient has a good constitution, and if the fever is not high, we may apply with even more success some bed steam baths, or foot steam.

If the fever is high, we give every day two or three half baths, 90° F., followed by a pour on the upper back and throat. These baths decrease the fever and prepare the skin for a profuse perspiration. Further, they draw the blood from the endangered mucous membrane to the surface of the body. It is evident that by these proceedings we satisfy also *number three,* especially when there is a steady, good ventilation, and the patient is given only a mild fluid diet of cooling fruit juices.

By following the above directions we will have prevented the most serious kinds of diphtheric processes. Nevertheless, if they appear in a slight way, we must also apply local treatment. This is done by deep gargling every hour with lukewarm water, mixed with a few drops of lemon juice, or if that causes pain, by mouth baths. Not less important are cool packs around the neck, as in picture.‡

In the beginning, these are to be renewed every forty or sixty minutes to reduce the inflammation;

*See Figure No. 21.
†See Figure 18.
‡See Figures 19 and 20.

later, a little warmer, and only changed every two
or three hours to better expel the products of decomposition.

Diphtheria treated in the above way seldom ends
fatally.

ECZEMA.

Eczema is an inflammatory excreting process in
the skin without putrefaction.

Its causes are either chemical or mechanical irritations, or internal diseases, as rickets, chronic catarrh
of the stomach, *scrofulousness*, etc. In most cases
it is sufficient to put rice powder on the attacked
place, and cover it with a thin piece of lawn or gauze.
In order to remove the excretion, wash it quickly, or
pat it with absorbent cotton dipped in warm water,
dry it with cotton as well, and let it dry by the air.

When scabs are formed, soften them by patting
them frequently with sweet oil. With this almost
dry treatment you have more success than with
much bathing and packs. When the scaling-off period
has begun, you may give patient sometimes short
tub baths of 85° F. to reduce inflammation. No soap
to be used.

EPILEPSY.

This nervous disease consists of an attack of unconsciousness, and in most cases of contractions of
the muscles. Its cause is unknown, but a tendency
to it is often inherited.

Overwork, grief, fright, worry, gluttony, self-abuse and anæmia favor an attack. The attacks often come unexpectedly; sometimes the patient feels its approach.

The pupils of the eyes are wide and do not contract when light strikes them. The face grows pale first, then purple. Some patients fall into a long sleep after the attack, and others soon grow conscious again.

This dreadful disease can either appear in connection with other diseases, as *scrofulousness,* nose and ear catarrh, worms, etc., or it comes as an independent disease.

In the first case, treat the disease which caused the attacks. In the latter case, do the following: During the attack do nothing but prevent the patient from hurting himself; after it is over, give him a refreshing, cool, sponge bath, and cold compresses on the forehead for headache.

Between the attacks, treat the patient thus: Give him every day either a hot foot-bath of fifteen minutes, followed by a cold wash-off of the whole body, or a foot vapor.

Further, give him every day a general and forehead massage.

His bowels must move daily. If constipated, cause evacuations daily by enemas and a diet of whole wheat bread, breadsticks, prunes, boiled figs, bonnyclabber, etc.

He ought to have at each meal only one-half as much as he would like to eat, and he should be induced to masticate all his food well and slowly, four times as long as he has been doing.

Coffee, tea, alcoholic drinks, sweets, cocoanut, all medicines, meats and fried food should be avoided.

Some epileptic people have a ravenous hunger almost all the time. Do not let them eat all day long, but give the patient a scanty meal at regular times, and an apple, an orange, or some other fruit between meals. This must be strictly adhered to, otherwise he will *never* become well.

Many a patient has an attack when he thinks of something sad or worrying. Such a one must be trained to use all his will-power, never to let such thoughts get hold of him, but to discard them immediately, and recall in their stead the very bright, funny or joyful events of his life. It is wonderful how this works.

I had several patients who could thus prevent an attack, even when they felt it coming upon them, and they grew quite well.

Keep everything sad or gloomy away from the patient, and let only bright, joyful influences surround him.

Fresh air, day and night, and much out-of-door exercise, besides gymnastics every morning and evening.* Air-baths and water treading tend greatly to a prompt recovery.

*See Figures 3, 4, 6, 11 to 16.

FAINTING.

Fainting comes with most heart diseases, hysteria, great pain, loss of blood, overwork, bad air, fear, fright, weakness, etc.

Put the patient in a horizontal position, loosen all tight clothes around the neck and waist, wash his face lavishly with cold water, rub his neck and chest gently downwards. If these measures are not effectual, dash a glass of cold water into his face.

Then treat regularly the disease which caused him to faint.

FALL, CONCUSSION OF THE BRAIN.

Keep continually cool compresses on the patient's head and give him directly a tepid 85° F. enema, and every hour a remaining enema of cold water. Further, give the patient a tub bath of 85° F., in which you rub his legs and arms thoroughly upwards; chest and back downwards, but no longer after his armpits have grown cool.

Then give him a chest and back pour of 70° F., and put him to bed with a hot-water bag to his feet, and a cold compress on his head. Repeat bath after two hours. If patient vomits and can swallow, give him often a teaspoonful of cold water. The diet must be mild and spiceless.

FEVER.

Formerly fever was regarded as a disease; not so any more. We now regard it as a symptom of a disease, and a healing factor. As this has been explained before, I shall not repeat.

One main symptom of fever is that great masses of products of decomposition enter the blood, and thus by its circulation, being carried to all parts of the body, they endanger life. A quickened heart action, causing perspiration and transpiration, as well as the excreting abilities of kidneys and lungs, will bring relief if great products of decomposition are not created in the sick body by wrong diet. By a "wrong diet" we mean all animal food, because at the time the animal is being killed there are products of decomposition—urea, xanthine, etc., in its body, which, entering the patient's digestive organs, demand for their digestion an increased action of heart, kidneys and blood-vessels. A healthy person may notice this in his own body, for after eating a good portion of meat he will feel his heart acting much quicker than after having eaten vegetables, fruit and cereals. Therefore, no feverish person should be given any animal food, except milk and eggs. A vegetarian diet does not bring into our bodies products of decomposition, neither do milk nor eggs. In order to keep up the resistive power of the body it is best, and the patient's instinct says the same, to give him especially fruit juices, cold soups,* cooked fruits, cereals, etc. If it is a case of prolonged fever, it would be advisable to add to the above some legumes—purée of peas or beans, almond milk and green vegetables.

Have the windows open day and night.

*See Chapter on "Hygienic Cooking."

FLATULENCE.

Flatulence indicates either an acute or chronic disturbance of the digestion caused by certain things we have eaten, as cabbage, kale, legumes, cakes, beer, etc., or a sedentary life. It may be caused by abdominal diseases, catarrhal condition, indigestion caused by no or too little mastication of food, hysteria, sores, etc.

Masticate the food well and slowly; avoid the above-named dishes; take abdominal and calf packs every night, or if a bad case, at night, and two each day, of two hours in length.

If it came with a cold, put vapor compresses on patient's abdomen, or apply a large hot-water bag.

Further, give the patient enemas for regular evacuations, and massage of the digestive organs, besides exercises "pull the branch," "sitting up," "head turning,"* and "picking up pebbles," page 54.

FLUX. (See DIARRHŒA.)

GALL-STONES.

Sometimes people have gall-stones without suffering from them, even if they are so large that you can feel them from the outside. At other times they signify a serious disease, with great pain in attacks of colic. This pain is caused by the gall-stones passing through the gall ducts and coming in contact

*See Figures 3, 5, 6.

with an obstacle. The pain comes generally very suddenly a few hours after a meal, and is felt mostly in the stomach, and in the right side of the abdomen. It is seldom confined to these places, but extends into the back, shoulders, right arm, and sometimes even into the legs. The abdomen is swollen and the liver very painful to the touch. Sometimes the patient has chills, is delirious and vomits. The pulse is irregular.

This disease attacks women more frequently than men—three times as often—because the women lace, and lead a more sedentary life.

In order to find out whether there are gall-stones, notice all the symptoms and search the fæces for at least a week, by putting them in a sieve and dissolving them in warm water. Thus you sometimes find the stones, sometimes only pieces, or none at all, if the stone has passed back into the gall-bladder.

The treatment must be a general one and a symptomatic one. The best means to relieve the pain is a hot sitz bath or half bath of 105° to 110° F. These reduce the pain, but in some cases vapor compresses put on the liver relieve it even more. These measures not only relieve the pain, but the heat causes a relaxing of the painfully contracted muscular walls of the gall-bladder and ducts, thus helping an easier passing of the gall-stones towards the intestines. Hot enemas help to relieve the pain.

At symptoms of collapse, conquer weakness by gently rubbing the patient with damp cloths.

After the attack, the patient must take regular

8

treatment as follows: Daily, two or three enemas of a pint or so of warm water, 75° F., followed after evacuation by a 60° F. remaining enema. These alone cause a freer flow of bile, consequently the moving of the obstacle—the accumulation of bile. The appetite increases, the urine shows less bile and the fæces look more normal.

Then give the patient every day a cold sponge bath, followed by moderate friction, which lessens the itching and sometimes banishes it entirely.

Also give the patient every day from two to four sitz baths, 85° to 90° F., from forty to sixty minutes each.

These baths improve the action of the bowels, the excretion of bile, the appetite, the urine, and remove headache and sleeplessness, and prevent an over-filling of bile in the blood.

The diet must be a mild one and not highly seasoned—oatmeal, toast, green vegetables, fruits, lettuce, bonnyclabber, almond milk, fruit soups, etc. Exercises "pull the branch," "sitting up" and "head turning,"* every few hours, if possible, help greatly to a prompt recovery.

A continued diet with fruit acids, and some onions daily, prevent the formation of new stones.

GONORRHŒA.

Gonorrhœa is nearly always caused by infection during intercourse with a person who has the dis-

*See Figures 3, 5, 6.

ease. It is an inflammation of the mucous membrane of the urethra caused by the transmission of gonorrhœa pus by the infecting person.

In order to prevent the infection take immediately after the intercourse several long (forty-five to sixty minutes) sitz baths, of 85° F. Then put on a T-tie. This tie consists of a piece of linen in the shape of a T. Wring it out in cold water; fasten the upper part around your waist and the lower broader part between the legs, with special six- to eight-fold rags around the penis. Put over the whole a T-tie of flannel, wear it all night and day, renewed during the day every three or six hours, followed by a wash of affected parts or by a sitz bath. This pack and the sitz baths draw out the poison and prevent the infection.

Women should rinse the vagina frequently with "Stamm's Vagina Cleaner," and take the above-mentioned sitz baths. A plain vaginal syringe does not do the work so effectually as the "Cleaner."

Rest as much as possible.

Do not drink coffee, tea, or alcoholic drinks.

Continue two to four sitz baths, and wear the T-tie day and night until cured.

Strong people may take two or three vapor-baths a week also, as they help to bring the poison out of the system.

Any time the T-tie grows too hot or uncomfortable it is to be renewed.

With this treatment the acute as well as the chronic gonorrhœa will be cured.

GOUT.

Gout is a diseased condition of the whole body, caused by an incomplete change of matter through a wrong way of living, especially too rich a diet and want of out-of-door exercise.

The first symptom is generally a great pain in the big toe of one foot during the night. The toe is red, hot and swollen. The patient is feverish with an increased pulse. The pain grows less towards morning.

Sometimes there is only one acute attack, but in chronic gout generally several joints are attacked quite frequently. In the course of time the joints grow more and more disfigured by deposits of uric acid.

There is also a gout of the skin, of the bowels, and a cartilage gout.

Acute gout and chronic gout of the joints can be cured if the patient is willing to change his mode of life, provided there are no serious organic diseases connected with it, although the disfigured joints can never be made normal again, but can be much improved.

For an acute attack of gout put the leg with the attacked foot in a horizontal position, wrap lower leg in warm cotton and put some hot-water bags or heated bricks around it. If the patient can stand damp heat give him either hot foot-baths, vapor compresses on paining foot, or vapor foot-baths.

When thus the attack of the first night is passed,

give the patient next day frequent vapor compresses, or increasing (in heat) hot foot-baths, and between these, foot packs. Continue this treatment for three or four days until you feel sure no attack will recur.

After acute attacks are thus averted treat their cause—the chronic gout. The treatment is the same as that for rheumatism.

GRIPPE (Influenza).

This disease is a feverish cold.

Every day take two or three half-baths, 90° F.

Day and night take trunk packs changed every two hours, and foot packs changed every four hours, followed each time by a sponge bath of 70° F. During the night the packs need not be changed unless the patient grows restless.

Give him two or three enemas, and six remaining enemas daily.

Let the patient gargle frequently with lemon juice and water.

If the fever is not high give him also some vapor-baths or dry sweats. (See figure 30.)

No solid food or animal food must be taken while the fever lasts; give him fruit juices and almond milk.

Let him have plenty of fresh air day and night.

HEADACHE.

This, in most cases, is the symptom of a disturbance in your body, or of a disease, and disappears with the cure of them.

When no cause for it can be found, as a cold, stomach trouble, constipation, anæmia, etc., it is generally of a nervous kind. Overworked people should take a rest.

With a sick headache, fast a few days; take stomach and calf packs, besides plenty of outdoor leisure walks, or garden work.

Avoid all alcoholic drinks and smoking.

If the head is very hot and the feet cold, take hot foot-baths and practice water treading to regulate your circulation.

For a habitual nervous headache, take a regular course of nerve treatment, and you will be cured. If you cannot have that, do the best you can by changing your wrong way of living to a hygienic one and apply the nerve packs. (Figures 24, 25, 26, 27.)

With any organic trouble, treat the affected organ and the headache will disappear.

HEART TROUBLE (Valvular).

Valvular heart disease, in most cases, is the outcome of an inflammation of the heart, causing either a contraction of the blood vessels in the heart, or enlarging of the holes, so that the valves cannot close; or contractions of the valves themselves.

The symptoms are so various, according to which valve or vessel is affected, that it would lead too far to describe them. Irregular circulation, shortness of breath when mounting stairs, etc., congestion in other organs, are regular occurrences, if compensation in the form of the thickening of the heart muscles does not take place.

Valvular heart trouble, if curable, can only be cured by the natural healing power in the patient's own body, assisted and stimulated by a strictly hygienic way of living, scientifically applied heart massage, and a diet consisting mainly of fruits, green vegetables and nuts. No alcoholic drinks, tea, coffee, flatulent dishes, soups or medicines. Increase the number of meals, but eat little at a time.

You should have an evacuation every day by eating much fruit and whole wheat bread; or if necessary, by enemas.

Avoid all excess in exercise; no running, jumping or even quick walking up an incline. There should be no bicycle riding, dancing, swimming, etc.

Indulge daily in walking on even ground, and in gymnastic exercises. Those indicated in illustrations are very helpful when executed without haste.*

Tepid half baths of short duration and sponge baths are very beneficial, but must be applied by a second person.

During the greater part of the year live at a shady place in the mountains and take level walks in the neighborhood. Spend all of your time out-of-doors.

HEART TROUBLE (Nervous).

This disease is treated the same as Angina Pectoris.

*See Figures 3, 4, 6, and 11 to 16, inclusive.

HÆMOPHILIA.

This is a kind of scorbute. It is in the whole system, with much inclination for bleeding, which is sometimes difficult to stop on account of the wrong composition of the blood, which makes it hard to coagulate. Profuse bleedings occur sometimes after an insignificant cause, like pricking the gums with a toothpick, a slight scratch, etc., on account of the weakness of the arterial walls.

The first thing to do, therefore, is to make the walls of the arteries strong and to create healthy blood. As the blood is poor in lime, and overfilled with carbonic acid, the diet of the patient should contain much lime and natron (soda).

These we have especially in raw and steamed green vegetables and juicy fruits. Besides this, the patient should take as little salt with his meals as possible, because it irritates the walls of the arteries and it creates an artificial thirst—thus watery blood.

To improve the blood still more, the patient should be much out of doors, take sun-baths and air-baths. Cold sponge baths and tub baths of 90° F., lasting five to eight minutes, taken every day, improve the capillaries. Gentle massage and moderate exercises should also be taken daily.

HAIR FALLING OUT.

The hair comes out through various causes, as after typhoid fever, skin diseases, etc. Worry and nervousness will also make it come out.

The main thing to stop its coming out is frequent washing of the scalp, with gentle backward rubbing. Hygienic living aids in retaining the hair, because it creates good blood.

Wear no head covering, or a very light one.

Do not worry, and masticate your food slowly.

HEMORRHAGE.

Hemorrhage is a flow of blood from the body. If the hemorrhage comes with a cough, then it usually is from the lungs; if vomited, from the stomach. Blood from the lungs is generally of a bright red color and foamy; from the stomach, it is dark.

If it is from the *lungs,* undress the patient and put him to bed.

Calm and console him by saying that there is no danger for him, even if another hemorrhage should occur.

Tell him to keep quiet and give him a glass of salt water to drink.

If the bleeding is very profuse, encumbering the air-pipes, so that there is danger of suffocation, command the patient to cough hard, though it may renew the bleeding.

Draw the blood from his lungs by putting pack of 70° F. on his abdomen, arms and calves of legs, re-

newed every twenty or thirty minutes. At the same
time put his hands into hot water, as hot as he can
stand. To his feet put a hot-water bag.

If, by the patient's indications, you know about the
place in the lungs from which the blood comes, put a
vapor compress on the same. Heat makes the blood
coagulate quickly and thus the blood-vessels are
closed.

In order to prevent coughing, give the patient
honey or the yolk of an egg with sugar stirred into it,
or cool water with raspberry juice.

The diet must be a fluid one of low temperature.

A *hemorrhage* from the *stomach* requires methodic
treatment.

Put the patient to bed, and let him stop all work.

The diet is of the greatest importance. It should
consist only of fluids, as buttermilk, clabber, sweet
milk, lemonade, almond milk, huckleberry wine or
some acid red wine boiled with sugar. By the contracting quality of these drinks we can often prevent
a recurrence of the hemorrhage.

After ten days the patient may eat some very well-
cooked rice, oatmeal, barley, milk toast, apple sauce,
and very soft green vegetables. All animal food
should be avoided during the acute state. All food
should be given in small portions and masticated
until it forms a fluid in the mouth.

Give the patient a sitz bath, 90° F., for twenty minutes, three times a day. Between times give him
stomach packs, 78° F., renewed every two hours, and
calf packs, renewed every four hours.

If he is constipated, give him once or twice a day an enema, 70° F., followed after evacuation by a remaining enema.

After the acute state is over, the treatment has to continue for some time, and the patient should continue to live in a hygienic way in order to prevent a relapse and the formation of cancer.

Hemorrhages from the *womb* are stopped by hot douches and internal (Thure Brandt) massage, besides rest. Nothing hot should be eaten.

HYSTERIA.

Hysteria is an irritation of the nerves, mostly through mental influences.

As all hysteric patients are more or less weak-minded, the physician can in many cases reach the best results by a spiritual influence as soon as he has gained the confidence of the patient.

Give him, or her, every day a cool or cold sponge bath and general nerve massage.

Hysterical contractions of the muscles are best cured by baths of 105° F., for ten minutes at the beginning, then increasing in length to forty-five minutes; then *very gentle* nerve massage.

When a bad attack occurs, give the patient a cold sponge bath, with gentle rubbing, or a half bath. For bad pains in the back or abdomen, apply local vapor compresses.

Much outdoor exercise and cheerful surroundings, cheerful books and practical training to use his will power, will help the patient to a prompter recovery.

INFANTILE PARALYSIS.

This disease usually comes suddenly, and with children between their first and fourth years.

Sudden high fever, pain in the head and limbs, with unconsciousness, are frequent symptoms. Later on, lameness of certain muscles follows, which is either temporary or lasting. If the latter, it can be prevented, in most cases, by a systematic course of Nature Cure treatment.

Wash the patient with cold water from the feet upwards; then give him a spinal pack, 80° F., and abdominal and calf packs, 85° F., renewed every two or three hours. Besides these, give him three times a day a half bath of 80° F. or 85° F., followed by a back-pour and frequently a gentle kneading massage of the extremities. Try to prevent lameness by frequent careful gymnastic exercises or by passive motion of the limbs.

Move the bowels by enemas of 70° F.

After the worst state is over you may give the patient a spinal pack every two hours, and twice a day a half bath of 93° F. for five to eight minutes.

When the symptoms of lameness have begun to disappear you may allow the patient to walk about a little, decrease the packs, but continue the massage, gymnastics and baths.

To prevent another attack, send the patient to a Nature Cure sanitarium as soon as he can get there without difficulty.

INFLAMMATION OF THE BRAIN.

This disease may be caused by a hurt, an inflammation near the brain or a diseased brain. Its main symptoms are severe headaches, numbness, delirium and chills and fever.

Put the patient to bed with his head rather high, on a soft horsehair pillow.

In order to draw the blood away from the head give the patient in the morning, at noon and in the evening, daily, a half bath of 85°-90° F., for ten or fifteen minutes. Numbness in the head, stiffness in the neck or pain should not prevent these baths. If the pains are *exceedingly* great, substitute for the baths cold sponge baths. When the seriousness of the symptoms has decreased, give the patient, day and night, throat packs and trunk packs, renewed every two hours, and calf packs, renewed every four hours. Should they dry sooner, renew them at once. At each removal wash the packed parts with cold water. After three or four days the packs can stay on during the night.

By the intestines we can draw the blood from the brain by several cool, small enemas, followed after evacuation by cold remaining enemas.

These treatments have to be strictly continued until the patient has regained consciousness, or until the gravest symptoms have passed. Then you may decrease the baths to two; then one daily. Give the packs only twice a day and during the night.

If the patient has a stiff neck, remove stiffness by

a gentle massage. Keep a cold compress on his head until he has no more headache.

The room must always be well ventilated, and the diet must be mild.

Do not use an ice bag on the head or neck; it increases the inflammation and the suppuration.

INTESTINAL INDIGESTION.

Follow the same treatment as for Diarrhœa.

ITCHING.

Itching appears often as a symptom of a disease, and disappears with the cure of the same. If it is of a nervous nature, give the patient long hot baths, or vapor baths followed by trunk and calf packs. You may also give him regular air-baths and sun-baths. Let his diet be very mild.

LUMBAGO.

Follow the treatment given for Neuralgia.

LUNG TROUBLE.

Follow the treatment given for Consumption.

MASTITIS (Sore Breasts).

In slight cases of mastitis wash the breasts from two to four times daily with cold water; bending over the basin, splash the water over the breasts;

then may follow a gentle circular rubbing of the same.

In serious cases, accompanied by great pain, put every two or three hours a compress of 85° F. on the breasts and hold them up with a suitable bandage.

Hot tub baths, rising from 95° to 110° F., for thirty to forty minutes; a vapor bath, followed by a trunk bath, 90° F., or vapor compresses on the breasts, are healing factors, and in most cases prevent an operation.

MEASLES.

Measles is an acute infectious disease.

In summer time the patient can be out-of-doors or in the garden all day long, except during the fever.

The windows must be opened day and night; the room a little darkened, according to the sensitiveness of the patient's eyes. Keep the temperature of the room in winter 60° F.

Both doctor and nurse should approach the patient only in white or light-colored clothes, as they attract less of the poison than the dark ones. They should be well shaken afterwards in the open air, to free them from the airy, gaseous, chemical poison. The nurse should gargle frequently with cold water, 80° F., and draw some up her nostrils to keep resistive the mucous membrane of the nose and throat.

Give the patient in the morning, at noon and at night a half bath, eight inches deep, of water, 10 degrees lower in temperature than that of his body.

These baths refresh the patient, ameliorate the catarrhal conditions, prevent their increase and make the skin able to put out the measly poison more profusely. After the fever has passed its height, two baths every day are sufficient.

In order to draw the blood from the mucous membrane, and to produce a better excretion of the poisonous gases, give the patient a trunk pack every two hours, along with a throat pack; every four hours give a foot pack, each followed by a short cool wash of the packed parts.

After the fever has almost or entirely gone, give the patient, according to his constitution, once or twice a day, a hot bath and a dry pack, followed by a tepid bath, 90° F., because the perspiration will bring out the poison so much more thoroughly than any other measure. Especially should this be done where the eruption of the measles is not profuse. The beneficial effects of these sweats is directly visible in the improved catarrhal conditions.

To this general treatment we have to add a local one in order to prevent bad after-effects. To this end the patient ought to gargle frequently with tepid water; his mouth, nose and ears should be cleansed often with soft, clean, wet cloths or absorbent cotton.

Diet as directed under "Fever."

Every morning give the patient a small tepid enema, even if he has had an evacuation, as it helps to lower the fever and to free the body from its poison.

As the patient grows better he can take fewer treatments.

Measles treated in the above manner will never leave any bad effects or cause "secondary diseases."

MELANCHOLY.

Give the patient every day a tub bath, 90° F., or a cold sponge bath; once a week a three-quarter nerve pack, and once a week a sweat, or bed steam bath.

Long and frequent leisure walks, sleeping with open windows, pleasant company, breathing exercises, a mild diet, enemas and general massage with special abdominal massage are of great benefit in this trouble.

With a strong will-power the patient must banish all grief and sorrow and cultivate cheerful, pleasant thoughts. Diversion in the form of traveling, picnics, excursions, etc., with cheerful company, is of great moment.

NERVOUS DYSPEPSIA.

This disease is a nervous stomach trouble.

Of the greatest importance is your influence upon the mental condition of the patient. As nervous dyspepsia is easily and thoroughly cured by Nature Cure treatment, tell the patient that he does not suffer from an incurable disease of the stomach, but that this organ is quite able to digest any food. To prove this, and to relieve him of his fear, let him eat anything he wants, as a test.

Insist upon thorough mastication of any food, and

let his meals be moderate in amount. Positively forbid the use of tobacco and alcoholic drinks.

Do not allow him to perform any brain work and but little manual labor.

To strengthen the body, give him every day a general massage, combined with a special organic massage of the stomach and abdomen.

Give him every morning a cold sponge bath, after which he goes back to bed for ten or fifteen minutes.

Give the patient alternately one evening a sitz bath, 90° F., twenty minutes' duration, and the next evening a tub bath, 90° F., for ten minutes.

Abdominal and calf packs during the night, and in very bad cases twice during the day, with air-baths and barefoot walking, prove very beneficial.

NERVOUS PROSTRATION.

Nervous prostration usually comes on by degrees, either from overwork, incessant grief, worriment, over-excitement, loss of sleep, excess of intercourse, anæmia, or the excessive use of alcohol and tobacco.

Its symptoms are mental and bodily fatigue, fitful moods, restlessness, both when asleep and awake; fear, irritability, and very often a giving out of the digestive organs.

Its prevention is easy if the patient is wise enough to stop its cause or causes in time.

When fully developed, the treatment is the same as that for neurasthenia. First of all remove the cause. If overworked, take a complete rest; discard tobacco, alcoholic drinks, coffee and tea.

In the beginning take a general nerve massage and a nerve pack every day. Later on an occasional bed steam-bath, or dry pack instead of the nerve pack, followed by a general massage.

Take two leisurely walks every day. Sleep with open windows.

Masticate your food very thoroughly.

Morning and evening take a long air-bath.

Cultivate cheerfulness in thought and seek cheerful society. Avoid worriment of every kind. Practice deep breathing at all times. Do not wear any heavy underwear.

NETTLE-RASH.

Its causes may be scratching with the nails during diseases which cause an itching of the skin, as jaundice, diabetes, etc. Sometimes it is caused by certain things we eat, or by nervousness, etc.

Take trunk and calf packs, renewed every two or three hours, followed twice a day by a bath of 90° F., the other times by a cool sponge bath.

In chronic cases add an occasional vapor-bath.

NEURALGIA.

Sometimes its cause is found in a cold, in constipation, anæmia, poor circulation, inherited tendency for it, poisoning, brain diseases, direct hurting or wounding of a nerve, etc. Sometimes we cannot find a cause. If you find the cause, remove it by a hygienic way of living and regular Nature Cure treatment.

Apply heat either in the form of vapor compresses or vapor-baths, and hot baths from 95° F., increased to 108° or 110° F., thirty to sixty minutes long.

Between times pack the painful parts in cool 77° F. packs.

If the patient does not like damp heat, treat him with dry heat—hot air-baths, hot sand-baths, wrapping painful parts in hot cotton, etc.

Besides these, give the patient very gentle stroking massage of affected part or near it if it cannot be borne on painful place. By degrees increase depth of stroking massage and go to kneading massage, by which poisons and obstacles in circulation will be removed and pain decreased.

NEURASTHENIA

Is treated in the same way as nervous prostration.

NEURITIS.

Neuritis consists in most cases in inflammation of the sheath of the nerve. It may be caused externally through a fall, strain, contusion, etc.; internally by an inflammation in the neighborhood of the nerve spreading to it.

Apply packs to ailing part, 60° F., renewed every two or three hours, and bathe it frequently in 80° F. water, besides a nerve pack every second day. For great pains give hot baths to painful parts, and rub the arms gently upwards twice a day.

NOSE BLEEDING.

A slight bleeding does not need any treatment. If it is profuse, put cold compresses on the forehead and nose of the patient. Cold pours over the neck and chest are helpful.

Further, let the patient draw up into his nose water mixed with lemon juice, or vinegar if lemon be not handy.

With very profuse bleedings the patient must go to bed with head very high; keep quiet, and avoid coffee, tea and alcoholic drinks.

If all this does not stop the bleeding, you have to ask a physician to apply Bellocq's tube.

OBESITY (Stoutness).

Many different medicines and treatments have been recommended for obesity, most of them more or less harmful.

We would treat the patient as follows:

People who have the habit of eating a great deal ought to decrease the amount.

Avoid starchy food, sweet things, fat and fluids as much as possible.

Do not drink anything at your meals, nor for half an hour before, nor two hours afterwards. In order not to create an artificial thirst, refrain from much salt and much spices.

Eat much fruit, green vegetables and nuts.

Take once or twice a week a mild vapor-bath or sweat, followed by a tub bath of 90° F., five or ten minutes. On days between take a cold sponge bath in the morning.

Twice or three times a day take physical culture exercises as described under "Physical Culture,"* ten to thirty minutes each, and two or three leisurely walks daily.

If possible, have a deep massage daily.

Take regularly the air-baths every morning and evening as long as possible, and once a week a sun-bath if you can, or a hot sand-bath.

Practice breathing exercises regularly in the open air, as that is one of the main means for the improvement of the blood.

OBJECT IN EYE, EAR, NOSE.

If in the eye, take a little piece of tissue paper dipped in water, raise the eyelid under which the object is, and slur the tissue paper over the eyeball, thus washing the object away.

Children often put beans, peas, etc., into their ears or nose. In such cases never use any instrument, as a hairpin, etc., as it only pushes the object further in, and may hurt delicate parts, as the drum, besides making it harder to remove the object. Take a syringe, and direct its stream aside of the object, and the returning stream will wash it out easily.

*See Figures 3, 4, 6, 11, to 16.

OPERATIONS.

The health of mothers is the foundation of the health of nations. The alarming increase in female diseases needs arresting. And how can it be done? There has never been a time in which there was such a passion for cutting as now, and how many thousands and thousands of women are either killed or made nervous wrecks by it!

Fortunately in Nature Cure we have the means of curing almost all female troubles without an operation. We employ our hands instead of the knife by giving the patient Thure Brandt massage (internal). By this massage we produce a better circulation, decrease and remove cysts and swellings, loosen adhesions, replace the dislocated organs, contract a prolapsed vagina, bring morbid matter to absorption, soften and render elastic hard, contracted parts, etc., etc. In short we, without a knife, create normal conditions and functions again.

Why do not all gynæcologists use it? you will ask. Because they have not learned it. They have acquired a passion for cutting, and may have thought it "greater" to perform a bloody operation, although I think there is more merit in making a sick organ well again than in simply cutting it out.

The Thure Brandt massage is bloodless (and nearly always painless) surgery, orthopædy, illustrated here so well by Dr. Lorenz two years ago. He said: "Fifty years hence no surgical instrument will any more be used, except the subcutaneous needle.''

Besides the Thure Brandt massage we apply compresses, tampons, sitz baths, enemas, douches, packs, physical culture, according to the case. But as a prevention is still better than a cure, young girls and mothers ought to be taught how important the nursing of a baby is, because if it is not fed properly it may get the rickets, by which very often the pelvis becomes crippled and the female organs dislocated, consequently abnormal conditions during pregnancy and childbirth.

The cases in which an operation is inevitable are very few. Most can be avoided through hygienic living and Nature Cure treatment. The welfare of our nation demands that operations should be restricted to the few unavoidable ones, for never before has there been a time when so many people died through operations than now.

Instead of pessaries, curetting and cauterizing we bring the organ back to normal conditions by removing the cause of the disease, the venous engorgement, by regulating the action of the bowels, by curing the cold feet, by massaging the womb, which produces in it a good circulation, and soon normal conditions in size, position, etc.

Instead of searching for the cause of the frequent degeneration of the ovaries, cysts, there is generally a diet prescribed which will favor the disease. And afterwards they cut fresh young girls (who ought to live and enjoy life) in their most sensitive parts, castrating and making nervous wrecks of them. Even insanity is often the outcome of it. Would any man allow himself to be castrated?

What is done by medical physicians to prevent all these female troubles? Do they tell the mother not to squeeze her daughters, often mere children, into corsets, until the muscles of the back and the abdomen have become too weak, and until the congestion in the abdominal organs and its consequences have become chronic through the atony (debility) of the abdominal muscles?

The word "Doctor" means originally "Teacher," but how many physicians are the teachers of their patients? Very few.

PALPITATION OF THE HEART.

Palpitation of the heart is not a disease in itself, but a symptom of a disease in anæmia, fatty degeneration of the heart, inflammation of the heart and several other heart troubles, hysteria, nervousness, constipation, etc.

Look up and treat the causes as directed, and with the removing of the cause the palpitation will cease.

PERITONITIS.

Peritonitis is an inflammation of the peritoneum, with these symptoms: Chills and fever, loss of appetite, vomiting, thirst, irregular bowel action, either constipated or diarrhœa and pain. Although peritonitis is mostly the outcome or caused by another disease, it needs more urgent treatment than the disease causing it.

Give the patient directly trunk packs, changed every forty to sixty minutes. In case these should cause great pain in the abdomen, give him only chest packs. At the same time give him calf packs, renewed every three or four hours.

As soon as the inflammation has decreased the packs are changed less frequently.

Besides these, give the patient, three times a day, morning, noon and evening, a sitz bath of 87° or 90° F. Its duration depends upon the feeling of the patient.

If the patient is too sick or has too much pain to take the sitz baths, substitute them by half baths, 90° F., or sponge baths.

Twice a day give him an enema, and after the evacuation a remaining enema to decrease the inflammation.

The diet ought to be a fluid one, consisting of almond milk, lemonade, brown soup and apple sauce.

Encapsulated suppurations demand the same treatment and vapor compresses, besides careful massage in order to bring the pus to the surface and eruption (breaking out).

After thus having averted the first danger, we begin to treat the cause of the peritonitis, stomach and bowel trouble, ovarian, womb, kidney, liver, spleen diseases, etc., as well as scarlet fever, diphtheria, measles, vaccination, rheumatism, etc.

PILES.

Piles are caused by a local disturbance of the blood-vessels of the rectum. The blood accumulates, enlarges the blood-vessels and cannot flow off sufficiently. This can be caused by a sedentary life, constipation, diseased conditions in the neighborhood of the rectum, poor circulation, etc.

Treatment is as follows:

Moderation in eating and drinking. Do not drink except when real thirsty.

Leisurely walks and physical culture exercises,* and "pick up pebbles," page 54.

Do not sit on any upholstered seat, but on open (reed, cane) seats.

Take every night an abdominal pack and calf packs.

Mornings and evenings, water treading and a sitz bath of 90° F. or 80° F., forty to sixty minutes long, with hot water, 110° F., to the feet, followed by a walk of fifteen to twenty minutes.

Against the constipation take enemas, followed by remaining enemas, given also two or three times more during the day.

To prevent friction of several exterior piles, put cold wet absorbent cotton high up into the anus.

For an attack of great pain give the patient a sitz bath of 95° F., and pour more and more hot water to it until it is 110° F.

In case you have not a sitz bath, take a wash-tub, or even a large wash-bowl.

*See Figures 3, 4, 5 and 16.

Let the diet be a mild one, excluding coffee, tea and alcoholic drinks, as well as tobacco.

For a thorough cure, massage and regular gymnastic exercises are necessary.

Do not sit long on any upholstered seat, horse or bicycle.

PLEURISY.

Pleurisy is an inflammation of the pleura. It can appear independently or as the outcome of another disease. Slight cases cause no discomfort. More serious cases cause pain in the chest and a friction sound, heavy breathing, bluish lips, and the patient lies mostly on the well side. In most cases there is cough, and sometimes fever. Percussion shows which part is affected.

Never use an ice bag with pleurisy, because it causes inflammation and suppuration.

Never use iodine; it irritates and inflames the skin, but does no good in any way.

Do not consent to an operation, because it is not necessary, but treat the patient as follows, and you will see great results. In dry pleurisy:

Keep the patient in bed; ventilate the room all the time.

Give the patient a mild diet.

Keep his bowels open with enemas, and above all things keep his feet constantly warm.

Give the patient every morning and every evening a half bath of 90° F., ten or twelve minutes, followed by a chest and back pour of 80° F. water.

During the day give the patient an 80° F. trunk pack and 77° F. calf packs, renewed every two hours.

At night give him a lung pack, 77° F. and calf packs, 80° F., not renewed during the night, excepting when the fever is high and the patient grows restless in them.

If a bronchial catarrh is connected with it, let the patient gargle frequently during the day with water and a little lemon juice.

The damp or moist pleurisy is treated the same if there is little secretion, but if there is much we reduce it by a dry, moderate diet, page 41, and sweats or vapor-baths, as well as after the fever is gone, by massage.

The purulent pleurisy is treated by vapor compresses, four to six each ten minutes, morning, noon and night. The heat draws the pus to the surface, and in most cases it bursts through the skin of the chest. In very few cases an incision on the most elevated part is necessary.

If after the absorption of the secretion the chest is crippled, do frequent exercises of the arm (raising and circular) of affected side, besides physical culture exercises.*

Pleurisy treated in the above way is scarcely ever fatal, and if massage is used it leaves the body in a much better condition than any other treatment would do.

*See Figures 11 to 14.

PNEUMONIA.

Pneumonia (catarrhal) is an inflammation of the pulmonary vesicles. This dreaded disease, by which thousands of lives are sacrificed every year, has lost most of its appalling aspect when treated by Nature Cure.

It is treated in the same way as a bronchial catarrh, with the addition of sending the patient when cured for a month or two into the mountains or to a Nature Cure sanitarium to regain vigor.

Pneumonia (croupy). This inflammation of the lungs is treated as follows:

From 8 to 10 A. M., trunk and calf packs, followed by a cold wash of packed parts.

From 10 to 10.30, rest.

From 10.30 to 12.30, same packs, followed by a half bath (8 inches deep), 90° F., instead of a wash-off.

A cold enema.

From 1 to 3 P. M., same packs as first in the morning.

One-half hour's rest.

From 3.30 to 5.30 P. M., same packs.

Rest till 6 P. M.

At 6 P. M., a half bath, 90° F.

Rest till 6.30 P. M.

An enema at 6.30 P. M.

Rest till 8 P. M.

At 8 P. M., trunk and foot packs for the night. These packs need only be removed if patient grows restless in them; otherwise they stay on till 6 A. M.

During the day the patient has to gargle frequently.

After each evacuation give patient a remaining enema.

Let the diet be a mild one.

After the crisis is past, you may add a few mild vapor treatments, as foot steam bath, or a bed steam bath, or a dry pack (sweat).

POISONINGS, SORES, WOUNDS.

Why does a wild animal never die of blood poisoning? Because it keeps its wounds clean by licking them, and because it goes to the nearest spring or brook and bathes its wounds in it at regular intervals.

What is the best thing to do if one is bitten by a snake? Suck the wound and spit out the poison.

What does the natural healing power in our body do to conquer successfully blood poisoning, for instance, puerperal fever? It creates a profuse perspiration, which throws the poison out of the body by the pores.

In these few phrases we have the foundation of a natural treatment of wounds and poisoning. First of all, keep the wound clean; and secondly, prevent the absorption of harmful wound excretions by the lymphatics and blood vessels, as this is the cause of all blood poisoning.

The next thing is to bring to work a sucking power, which draws out the poison. That cannot always be the mouth, but in linen and cotton we have the means. It has been recognized as a fact by all advanced physicians that a wound which is continually covered with a wet compress cannot suck up harmful wound products. Any clean water will do, and the compress ought to be covered with a piece of flannel to prevent its too rapid evaporation, and to have it grow warm soon, as thus it draws the blood to the wound, which is necessary for a sufficient growing of tissue and for the quick excretion of the bad products of the wound.

Even if there be some foreign matter in the water, it does not matter, as it will stick to the damp cotton or linen. (People who believe in the antiseptic by carbolic acid or corrosive sublimate cannot understand this. They will, though, believe after having tried it once).

The compress ought to be thick enough to keep damp from four to six hours, after which time it is removed, and if necessary the wound and its surroundings washed with water of ordinary temperature, and the compress renewed with well-washed or fresh material.

As we cannot always be sure that the wound has not absorbed some infectious matter before this treatment began, it is necessary to do something else to prevent blood poisoning, because the blood poisoning takes place only when the infectious matter has reached the heart, and thus gets into the arteries. On the way we must try to catch it. This is done first by a pack of damp linen or cotton being wrapped around that part of the body which lies between the wound and the heart, covering it well with flannel. Change it like the compress every four to six hours.

If infectious matter was already absorbed there, it will show after several packs a rash, in the form of little pustules.

The effect of these packs is quite a different one from that of the compress. This latter sucks the poison directly out of the wound, while the former enlarges the pores of the skin by its damp warmth and draws much blood to it, thus causing a great perspiration and transpiration. In this way the poisonous gases are carried off by direct perspiration, and the other poisonous matter in the form of pustules.

Thus we bring about artificially the same process which the natural healing power of our body uses in acute skin diseases (scarlet fever, pox, exanthema, etc.).

If fever indicates that the poison has already entered into the circulation, we must put packs beside the above on most parts of the body, thus having millions of pores helping us to draw out the poison.

Never use ice on wounds, because it works against the circulation, and thus brings about mortification.

PUERPERAL FEVER.

Puerperal fever (childbirth fever). Put patient into a sitz bath of 90° F., with the feet in hotter water, for fifteen or twenty minutes, covered with a blanket in winter time. After this, put her to bed

10

with a hot-water bag to her feet, and a thick layer of wet absorbent cotton, 92° F., covered with flannel, at the vagina, renewed every hour or two, according to flow. Cold compress on the head, renewed every three minutes.

Keep her bowels open with enemas. Give her cool drinks of fruit juices, buttermilk and almond milk.

Keep the room well ventilated day and night at a temperature of 65° F.

Repeat the sitz bath three times a day till the fever is gone.

RASH.

A rash is noticed either as a symptom of an organic trouble, a feverish disease, or independently of either, from impure blood. In any case it is an endeavor of the natural healing power in our body to expel poisonous matter, and we ought to assist it in this effort.

Take daily a bed steam bath or a dry pack (sweat), followed by a tub bath of 90° F., five to eight minutes, or by a cold sponge bath.

Fast a day or two, and avoid all medicine, coffee, tea, alcoholic drinks, rich food, fried food, tobacco, sweets, etc.

Do not drink anything at your meals, and masticate all you eat *well* and slowly.

Take two long air-baths every day, and at least two leisurely walks or other out-of-door exercise daily with deep breathing.

Do not wear any close, heavy underwear, and discard a fur jacket or fur cloak.

Sleep with open windows. Do water treading mornings and evenings, besides exercises as directed under "Physical Culture."*

RHEUMATISM.

There are different kinds of rheumatism, inflammatory, acute and chronic rheumatism of the joints, and muscular rheumatism. Its causes are want of skin action, exposure, wrong diet, want of fresh air and exercise.

Man is the only animal suffering from a diathesis of uric acid. How is this? The greatest physicians of our time attribute it to a wrong diet, especially a meat diet. The proof of this they find in the urine, because when a man lives on a vegetarian diet there is no uric acid in his urine, or only slight traces, while when he lives on a meat diet there is found a daily amount of two grammes and more of uric acid in it. A person who has to cleanse his body daily of two grammes of uric acid is continually in danger of its precipitating and causing rheumatism. Therefore, we advise as a prophylaxis (prevention) of rheumatism and gout to refrain from animal food as much as possible.

The urine of carnivorous animals scarcely ever contains any uric acid, because their bodies are adapted to a meat diet, while the anatomy and physiology of a human body is adapted to a fruit, nut and

*See Figures 3, 4, 6, 11 to 16.

vegetable diet. Man cannot oxidize meat completely,
therefore it is brought in his digestive organs to a
state of incomplete digestion, namely uric acid. Dr.
H. Lahmann says about this: "Man cannot be
classed as carnivorous, and cannot eat flesh unpun-
ished."

Cereals and pulse produce also a great amount of
uric acid in a human body. We may eat those things
when well in a small quantity, but the main part of
our diet ought to consist of fruits, nuts and green
vegetables.

The precipitation of uric acid in our body causes
not only rheumatism, neuralgia and gout, but also
rheumatic joints, organic heart trouble and apo-
plexy.

A thorough cure for the above-named ailments
consists, therefore, first of all, in a change of diet.
Then, in order to cure the affected body, take every
day a partial or whole vapor-bath (according to
constitution and ailment), followed by scientific massage.

Painful joints are packed after the massage, to
soothe the pain and help the dissolving of the uric
acid in those places.

Weak persons take trunk and calf packs instead of
vapor-baths, with an occasional bed steam bath.

If constipated, take an enema every day, followed
by a remaining enema after the evacuation.

As soon as most pain is gone the patient, directed
by a physician, should begin gymnastic exercises that
will best benefit the ailing parts.

After the cure is complete the patient may eat meat once a day—white meat preferred.

If you cannot have massage, exercise afflicted parts frequently, especially after the sweats, baths and pack.

RICKETS.

Rickets is the outcome of a serious disturbance in the nourishment of the baby, consequently dissæmia (an abnormal composition of the blood), and finally a want of lime in the bones, with an abnormal excretion of lime salts.

It mostly appears in children during the years of teething.

The child's condition is first noticed when it cannot walk at the usual age, and when its teething does not progress properly. The mother calls in a physician, and he pronounces the trouble "Rickets."

Children nursed artificially get it more frequently than those nursed by their mothers. The wrong diet is one of the main causes.

The fresh air is very important, as housed-up children get this disease frequently, but scarcely ever does a child who leads an out-of-door life all the time.

Uncleanliness is another cause.

Sometimes the disease appears very gradually. The child is weakened by continued diarrhœa, cries much in the night and becomes feverish. In the morning you find it in a profuse, acid, bad-smelling perspiration. Motion and touch seem to hurt it.

After some time the bones of the child undergo a change, the joints enlarge so that people call them "double joints." The skull enlarges greatly, and almost in a square form, while the face seems to form a very small part of the head.

The skull openings remain open till the second or third year and soft at their borders.

The lower jaw is often deformed by the disease.

The chest is marked with the so-called "Ricket Rosary," two rows of button-like projections at the points where the ribs join the rib cartilage. Sometimes the sides of the chest are drawn in, thus forming the so-called "chicken breast."

The pelvis often grows deformed, and proves often in later life a great obstacle to a normal childbirth.

Treatment.—Nurse your child yourself. If impossible, do at least refrain from putting one-half or one-third of water into the cow's milk.

Give the child fruit juices and vegetables, as directed under "HEALTHY CHILDREN."

Keep the child in the open air most of the time, and let it sleep with open windows.

Do not put tight fitting clothes nor heavy, closely woven underwear on it.

Do not give it meat, wine, beer or cod-liver oil, candy, cakes or ice cream.

RINGWORM.

This is a contagious skin disease, mainly appearing in children and young boys, mostly on the head.

Cleanse the affected part well with pure soap and water.

Then give the patient frequent head baths of forty to sixty minutes' duration, 80° F.

In the night put a pack on affected part, followed by a gentle wash with absorbent cotton.

Then, after three or four days of thus cleansing the head, pull out all loose, sick hairs and wash those places several times daily with water with lemon juice in it.

Thus treated, it will be cured in six or eight weeks, especially if a hygienic way of living is observed at the same time.

ROSEOLA.

Roseola is treated the same as measles.

SCARLET FEVER.

Scarlet fever is an acute disease, mostly of children, and contagious, with a typical eruption of the skin. Its cause is unknown.

Treatment.—Put the patient to bed and keep him there till the scaling-off is over. At the end of this latter period he may pass a few hours out of bed every day, in summer time, even a little in the open air in a protected place.

School should not be attended before the eighth week is past; first, in order not to interrupt his convalescence, and secondly, to be able to do everything for the prevention of an inflammation of the kidneys.

It is necessary to follow for quite a while a mild diet, as nothing so much favors the development of an inflammation of the kidneys as the so-called "strengthening diet," consisting of meat, beef tea, wine, eggs, etc.

It is also of the greatest importance to make the patient gargle frequently with tepid water, and have his nostrils, mouth and ear passages often washed.

In the beginning of the sickness, and after the fever is gone, give the patient every day a hot bath, 105° F., for ten minutes, followed by a wash-off of 80° F. These baths prevent, sometimes, the scaling off of the patient's skin.

Give packs and diet the same as directed under Measles.

SCIATICA.

Sciatica is an inflammation of the sciatic nerve, from the hip downwards, rarely involving the spinal cord. Its causes are very various: exposure to cold, and dampness, hurts, constipation, diseases of the womb, tumors, inflammations, operations, etc.

On account of this, our first aim must be to remove the cause.

The pain is mostly in the hip and along the back part of the upper leg, although it may extend to the toes. As a rule the pain is constant, with severe attacks at intervals. In chronic cases, atrophy of the muscles and partial lameness may result.

At the time of a very painful attack apply vapor compresses, changed every ten minutes on painful points. These are followed by a wash of the affected parts, 80° F.

If the patient can sit, give him frequently a hot half bath, increasing from 95° F. to 110° F., or a foot steam, followed by a tub bath, 90° F.

If the patient cannot sit, give him frequently a bed steam bath, with hot bottles for legs and hips, followed by a cool sponge bath.

During the pauses between the painful attacks pack the hips of the patient in linen with 80° F. water.

Especially beneficial are massage and gymnastic exercises. They improve the circulation, substitute the wanted exercise, stretch the contracted nerve and prevent atrophy of the muscles.

After the sciatica is cured, the patient ought to harden himself systematically through cold sponge baths, cool 85° F. tub baths, sun-baths, sand-baths, air-baths, barefoot walking on damp, sunny lawns, and gymnastic exercises described under ''Physical Culture.''*

SCROFULA.

Scrofula is a blood disease in children. If it is not cured in childhood it grows later into consumption. Its causes are wrong diet, want of fresh air and uncleanliness. Its symptoms are enlargement and inflammation of the bones and joints, especially of the lymphatic vessels, skin diseases, catarrh of eyes and

*See Figures 3, 4, 11 to 16.

bronchials. The patient looks pale, puffed up, with enlarged head and abdomen.

Give the child a diet consisting mainly of fruits, nuts and green vegetables. No medicine or cod-liver oil.

Daily massage and physical culture to improve the change of matter.

Further, give him daily a tub bath of 85° F. or 90° F., ten or fifteen minutes, preceded twice a week by a steam bath or a dry pack (sweat).

On the swollen glands put packs of 75° F., renewed every three hours during the day.

Scrofulous eyes are washed six or eight times daily with absorbent cotton dipped into 75° F. water.

Between times, put day and night, every three hours, compresses of 75° F. on the eyes.

By hypertrophy and suppuration of the glands an operation can be avoided by applying twice daily four to six vapor compresses, renewed every ten minutes. In many cases these soon bring the swelling down. In other cases suppuration sets in quickly (three to eight days) and bursts under the vapor compress.

At the height of suppuration the patient often gets high fever and chills, which make the case look more dangerous than it is. The bursting of the glands greatly relieves the patient, and the further treatment of the glands consists only of packs.

Sometimes the case is prolonged by part of the glands remaining hard. These have to be softened by vapor compresses as the first were.

Scalds on the head are washed eight to ten times daily, with absorbent cotton and a pack put on between times.

The rash on the face and body are washed in the same way, dried with cotton and powdered with rice powder.

During the night put gloves on the child's hands to prevent its scratching.

If convenient give him some sand-baths too. ·

SELF-ABUSE.

This is a very bad habit—nay, a carnal vice—consisting in an unnatural satisfying of the sexual desire, causing mental and physical weakness, degeneration and often insanity.

Its symptoms are shyness, sullenness, inactivity. The person stays much alone, looks pale, grows thin in spite of a good appetite.

Here we can, better than in most cases, apply prevention, which is better than a cure, by refraining from frequent intercourse during pregnancy, as this creates an abnormal sexual lust in the child; by keeping the child away from bad companions, who might teach it this ruinous habit.

Further, let the child sleep alone; do not take it into your bed either, for the touch of its little hand to bare parts of your warm, soft body might be the first inducement to the habit.

In conversation and literature everything relating to the matter must be avoided.

If you raise it hygienically, it will probably never practice it.

But if once you notice him practicing this bad habit, do everything to stop it.

If old enough, talk to him seriously, and punish him if he continues, for here is a case where leniency is not love, but, on the contrary, will result in the total ruin of your child. There is no vice on the earth practiced so much as this, and causing so much ruin to humanity; it makes physical and mental cripples of men, and often leads to insanity.

Give the child a mild, spiceless diet, a light evening meal of soups (see chapter on "Hygienic Cooking,") cool baths, much out-of-door exercise, running, ball play, swimming, rowing, physical culture exercises, described under "Physical Culture,"* long walks, sleeping with open windows on a hard mattress, with not too heavy bed clothes.

If the habit has fully developed into a disease, give him nothing but whole wheat bread and fruit to eat for a time.

Bathe him twice a day in water of 75° F. or a sitz bath of the same temperature for twenty minutes.

Watch him day and night.

Put a trouser-nightgown on him at night, and go to his bed regularly two or three times during the night to uncover him to see where his hands are.

Do the above faithfully, and you will save your child from ruin.

*See Figures 3, 4, 5, 16.

Many a girl has come to me ruined by this dreadful habit, and cursing her mother for not warning her.

Do not allow your fate to be theirs, for you can and ought to prevent it.

Our "Law and Order Societies," which are so zealously endeavoring to abolish houses of ill-repute, would get more nearly at the root of the evil if they introduced into our school system classes for young girls and mothers, to teach them the prevention of an abnormal sexual passion in their offspring. For, as it is, those houses are a necessary evil to protect decent women from "almost madmen."

SLEEPLESSNESS.

If it comes as a symptom of a disease, it will disappear when the latter is cured.

If noise, pain or other circumstances interrupt your sleep, remove them, and you will sleep.

But if it comes from worry, sorrow, etc., you ought to use all your will power to put all anxious thoughts out of your mind, and think only of pleasant things—Nature's beauty, rippling brooks—and you will then say "I will now sleep long and well."

Avoid all rich, heavy food at your evening meal. Take a long air-bath and a cold sponge bath before retiring; or put at the back of your neck, upon some rubber sheeting (to avoid wetting the pillow) a cold wet towel; or take an hour's leisurely walk before retiring.

If you can have it, take a good, gentle nerve massage, which does much to induce sleep; take also abdominal and calf packs, or a long run before going to bed.

Sleeplessness in children is generally caused by disturbances in their digestive organs. An enema at night, followed by a stomach and calf pack, does wonders.

SMALLPOX.

Smallpox is a contagious skin disease.

There is no preventive for smallpox. Vaccination prevents neither smallpox nor death from it, which is proved by statistics of many great *"observing physicians."*

The natural healing power in our bodies shows the physician the way by which the poison ought to be removed from the body. It pushes the poison-laden blood with feverish heat into the skin, swells it, and pushes out of its openings (pores) the poison of the system. We ought not to suppress, but help this action of the sick body in the following way:

At the beginning of the disease it is very good to give the patient some hot baths, increasing from 100° F. to 110°, or 112° F., but no packs.

Later keep packs on the trunk and legs of the patient day and night, renewed every two hours, to draw the poison mostly to these parts and away from the face.

These packs promote such a quick removing of the poison that it has no time to eat deeply into the papillary tissue of the skin to cause scars, but remains on the surface, often not going to the face at all, but only to packed parts.

If it goes to the face put on it a mask of six or eight layers of old, soft linen, with holes for eyes, mouth and nostrils. Wring it out in cool water and keep it damp all the time by sprinkling water on it. This mask will prevent the scars in the face better than anything can do, for it draws the poison into the damp linen instead of letting it destroy the papillary tissue of the skin.

Gargle regularly with lemon juice and water; and keep the bowels open.

Diet as directed under "FEVER."

It is well to stop the packs when the scabs come off the pox, and take three or four times a day some absorbent cotton, dipped in cold water, and tip repeatedly the pox with it. Then tip them with dry cotton, and put rice powder on them.

Any secondary diseases are treated as directed under heading of the same.

SORES.

Look up "POISONING."

SORE THROAT.

Gargle every half hour with lemon juice and water, or take mouth baths with same.

Put a pack on neck, renewing it every three hours during the day; it can stay on all night if thick. If the feet are cold, take a hot foot bath or a foot vapor-bath twice a day.

Inhale vapor twice a day, too, for fifteen minutes, if it is a severe case, and take frequent mouth baths (page 196).

SPRAINED ANKLE.

Avoid all exercising of the foot, but treat it directly thus: Take a long strip of linen three or four inches wide, wring it out in cold water and wrap it around the ankle and middle of foot alternately in form of an 8. Then wrap over it in the same way a long strip of dry flannel. Put the leg in a horizontal position, and renew the pack every two or three hours during the day, but let it stay on all night. After removing the pack wash the ankle and foot with cold water, and if it is swollen rub it with the points of your middle fingers around the ankle bones in a circular way till the swelling is reduced. Then renew the pack.*

After the greatest pain is over let the patient begin to walk a little, increase exercising it systematically, even if it pains, for it prevents stiffening of the muscles and hastens the cure.

STRICTURE OF THE BOWELS.

A stricture may be caused by obstacles in the intestines in the form of great masses of fæces, gas, gall-stones, etc., or by outside pressure with a tumor, or after sores, through scars; and it may be caused by a dislocation of the bowels themselves.

*See Figure 18.

In most cases, there is much abdominal pain, difficulty in urinating, the abdomen is much enlarged, the circulation is poor, patient feels very weak, hands and feet grow cold, and his eyes sink low in their sockets.

First of all, if the stricture is caused by accumulation of fæces give the patient an enema of 95° F., in a lying or kneeling position. Let the water (one pint) run slowly, and after removing the syringe press his buttocks together to help him keep it pretty long, rubbing with the other hand at the same time his abdomen, left side, upwards and above the navel from left to right side, to bring the water up as high as possible.

After the evacuation give him a remaining enema.

Repeat these enemas till several profuse evacuations have passed.

Then give him a sitz bath of 90° F. at least twice a day, but if the pain continues give them hotter, up to 110° F., and between times abdominal packs or (if no inflammation) some vapor compresses.

In severe cases the patient must be nourished by enemas of almond milk only, till all danger is averted.

Afterwards, and in less serious cases, the diet should consist of milk, fruit, soups (see chapter on "Hygienic Cooking"), mush, lettuce and almond milk.

Give enemas and abdominal massage twice a day till a complete cure is effected.

If a dislocation of the womb is the cause, the organ must be brought back into normal place.

Tumors, as the cause, frequently demand an operation.

SYPHILIS.

Only reluctantly I write about this most dreadful disease, but the thought that so many thousands are not only themselves miserable from it, but that it is the ruin of whole families for generations, decided me to do my best in advising a prevention and a cure.

As I am not writing a text book, however, I will refrain from relating the history and different stages of the disease.

Syphilis is either inherited or gotten by infection, by a kiss, intercourse, water closet, drinking from vessels of syphilitic people, not thoroughly cleansed medical instruments, vaccination, etc., etc. Anybody can get it, and more than once.

The first symptoms of the infection appear only a week or two after exposure in the form of a hard knot or a sore. Then the lymphatic glands begin to swell.

Then pass again some weeks without change, during which the poison enters the blood and then produces sores on the skin and on the mucous membrane.

Sometimes the poison affects after this the bones and the inner organs.

At the second stage appear frequently fever and chills.

When the sores appear in the mouth and nose they

grow very troublesome with itching, burning, irritation and pain.

Sometimes the eyes, lungs, kidneys and spleen become affected, as well as the muscles and bones.

When the nervous system becomes affected the patient grows from bad to worse; lameness, headache, neuralgia, sleeplessness, epilepsy, St. Vitus' dance, insanity, are its consequences.

Formerly this dreadful disease was regarded as incurable, and for the suppression of its symptoms the physicians up to our time have mainly prescribed mercury, but this gives in almost all cases only a temporary relief, as there are always relapses; but mercury is a very poisonous medicine which does the body more harm than if the patient did not take any medicine, for it is the cause of very alarming secondary diseases, especially quite serious nervous diseases, kidney trouble, lameness, insanity, etc. Proof of this statement is that the peasantry, who are often infected by soldiers returning from war, and who do not use mercury, have none of these dreadful diseases in later life. Most heavy metals are dangerous poisons for the human body. By lead, certain groups of muscles are irreparably lamed; zinc causes spinal disease, and mercury destroys certain parts of the nervous system.

A prevention of this dreadful disease can only be aimed at successfully directly, or in a few hours after the infection, because the poison is still near the surface.

First wash off well the infected parts. According

to our explanation about the treatment of poisoning, we then wrap around the infected part a cold, wet rag three to six-fold, and over that, with three-fold flannel a T-tie, explained on page 115. Renew it every four hours, or before it is dry, wash off, and put the pack on again.

In the mornings and evenings of the next days take a sponge bath to stimulate skin action.

Ladies take a lukewarm douche, then they put a tampon*, with 95° F. (or cold) water into the vagina, and take it out after four hours, take another lukewarm douche and renew the tampon. Repeat this proceeding for two days and two nights, after which time two tampons every day and during the night for three more days will have drawn out the poison. In this way we are pretty sure to prevent the disease, as we have often seen during our practice.

A thorough cure of the developed disease takes three years of hygienic living, besides a regular course of Nature Cure treatment of eight to ten weeks, as follows:

Every second day take a vapor-bath, or if you cannot have that, a dry pack or sweat. Strong people take it every day for two weeks, then every second day.

Besides this, take every night a trunk pack and calf packs, followed by a cold sponge bath in the morning. Do this for ten weeks. During this time take a mild, dry diet to create new blood.

Take no meat, no sweets; but plenty of fruits, nuts

*See Figure 10.

and green vegetables. Tobacco and alcoholic drinks
must be avoided, and not more than half a pint of
fluid taken every day. If this treatment is tiring
or weakening the patient can stop it for a week and
take it up again. This treatment will in the beginning make the sores increase, which is necessary, as
it means an increased action of the natural healing
power in the body expelling the poison. After a
time the sores will decrease more and more, and
finally disappear entirely.

When the skin is normal again the patient should
have a daily general massage of twenty to forty
minutes, because it improves the change of matter,
which is of the greatest importance in all diseases.

In order to avoid a relapse the patient should
after these ten weeks of regular every second day
treatment, continue for several months longer the
night packs, and one or two vapor-baths every week.

For affections of the throat, gargle ten to twenty
times daily with lemon juice and water, or with
huckleberry juice and take mouth baths; further,
avoid all highly seasoned dishes and smoking.

For "Vitus" make first eye compresses of 65° F.,
change every thirty minutes.

When the acute inflammation is over give the eyes
twice daily a vapor-bath, followed by washes of 77°
F., water.

For the great nerve pains we apply quickly soothing vapor compresses, packs of those nerves and
massage.

Syphilitic people ought not to marry until entirely
cured.

TAPEWORM.

Sometimes people have a tapeworm without knowing it, but they find sometimes parts of one in their fæces, looking like pieces of tape.

In other cases there are these symptoms: pressure and pain in the abdomen, increasing after the eating of onions, herring, pickles, etc. Sometimes vomiting, diarrhœa, constipation, headache, itching of the nose and vertigo.

Its cause is: eating raw meat.

Fast eight or ten hours, then eat only either a salted herring or cranberry sauce and the crushed seeds of the pumpkin for several meals; take several enemas during that day, and watch your fæces for signs of the worm. For a complete cure the head of the tapeworm must come out. If it does not come by these enemas, take half a cup of sweet oil, followed soon by another enema. If this does not bring it, repeat the whole. It has never failed me after a second trying.

TEETHING.

The teething of a baby should take place without any discomfort to it. It is but natural that the gums should be hotter and redder than before teething; but when it grows feverish and an inflammation of the mouth appears, it shows that the child has not been nursed properly.

During teething, wash the baby's mouth often with

a clean, soft rag and cold water, and give it a hard crust of bread to bite on.

If the child has any fever or convulsions, give it every night an abdominal pack and calf packs, followed in the morning by a warm bath 90° F., pouring a pitcher of cool water on the upper part of its back before taking it out.

The main thing is wholesome food and fresh air day and night.

THRUSH.

Thrush is a mouth disease, consisting of deposits on the mucous membrane of the mouth, representing an exuberant growth of fungus.

Its most frequent cause is neglected cleanliness with babies' mouths.

Mild cases do not cause much discomfort, but serious cases are connected with diarrhœa, abdominal pain, etc. As a prevention, keep your babies clean and wash their mouths after every meal with a soft, wet rag. Further, keep the nipples of their bottles clean, and wash your breast after every nursing.

When thrush has appeared, wash the baby's mouth before and after every nursing with water mixed with a few drops of lemon juice.

If connected with diarrhœa, give it treatment as directed under same.

Bottles are most thoroughly cleaned with bread crumbs and cold water.

TYPHOID FEVER.

Its first symptoms are generally loss of appetite, headache, restless sleep, vertigo, pains in back and legs, a tired feeling, swollen spleen, and coated tongue.

Its cause is not always impure water, but often self poison, which attacks the intestines, in which it produces sores.

There is scarcely any case of it without fever. This rises gradually the first week, keeps on its height the second, and pretty much so in the evenings of the third, while in the mornings of the third it gradually grows lower. After that it decreases as gradualy as it rose the first week. There are differences from the above in slight cases. During the first week there appears generally a rash on the abdomen, chest and back. Constipation is generally from the first, sometimes changing to diarrhœa. The fæces are bright yellow; when standing form a low, crumbly, yellow sediment with a dim watery part over it.

Bronchial catarrh is a frequent symptom.

Pulse is from 90 to 120 beats.

Nervous affections, unconsciousness and delirium appear in almost all cases.

Bleeding from the rectum and perforation make typhoid fever almost always fatal.

All critical physicians are unanimous in their opinion that we have in water treatment the best results in typhoid fever, because it lowers the fever, nearly always prevents stupor of the brain, improves the appetite, improves the catarrhal conditions so that scarcely ever dangerous secondary lung diseases appear, retention of urine is prevented, the skin becomes more able to transpire and to perspire the typhoid poisons, bed-sores and perforation are prevented.

All this shows how manifold are the beneficial effects of a single healing factor of Nature Cure.

Treatment.—During the first and second week give the patient, according to fever and constitution, from three to six half-baths daily (eight inches deep) of 90° F., ten minutes, followed by pouring cold water over the chest and back of the patient. Dry him with mild rubbing and put him in bed again.

Besides these give the patient during the first three weeks every day (regardless of diarrhœa or constipation) four one-half pint 70° F. enemas, which are followed, after the evacuation, by a cool remaining enema each time.

Further, give the patient during the first three weeks of his sickness, trunk and calf packs to be changed every two hours (as described with measles) in the day time, but kept on during the night if the patient does not grow restless.

If the patient falls asleep during one of these packs, do not waken him for its renewal.

During menstruation the patient continues to take the enemas and packs, but instead of the baths we give her sponge baths, as this occurrence generally diminishes the dangerous symptoms. A moderate use of these baths is only necessary (also) during the menstruation if the fever has a dangerous height and secondary diseases have occurred.

A weak heart and stupor are no counter signs for the above treatment.

After the fever has decreased considerably, and even is entirely gone, we have to continue the above prescribed treatment, although only half of the packs, baths, etc., each day.

Of the greatest importance are also the hygienic-dietetic influences:

1. The room, always well ventilated, ought to be of a temperature of about 65° F.

2. The bed must be smooth. No feather beds.

3. If the patient be in a stupor, his mouth must be washed frequently with soft linen or absorbent cotton dipped in cold water. As he generally remains lying on his back, he must sometimes be changed to a side position.

4. To prevent bed-sores keep day and night a basin of fresh, cold water under his bed, underneath where he lies.

5. During the feverish period his diet must consist of fluids only, fruit juices, buttermilk, clabber, almond milk, cereal soups, etc. Later, milk toast, breadsticks, cooked fruits with little sugar and no seeds or peel. Even during the time of convalescence we have to use great precaution in the patient's diet, especially to return to mushy and solid food by *very slow degrees.*

6. In cases of great stupor, or accompanying

throat diseases, we have to feed the patient through the rectum by enemas of almond milk, which will nourish him satisfactorily.

7. If during stupor the urine is not discharged we have to take it with the catheter.

8. Should hemorrhage of the bowels take place we must keep the patient's body as quiet as possible, stop baths and enemas, apply only every thirty to sixty minutes tepid abdominal 70° F. compresses, some remaining enemas 65° F., besides sponge baths.

With the above treatment I have never lost a typhoid fever patient.

UREMIA.

Its cause is poisons of the organism entering the blood because the kidneys are not able to expel them.

Slight cases begin with a headache, restlessness, oppression, sleepiness, fear, belching and temporary lameness.

Serious cases begin with vertigo, bad headache, cold and numbness, besides pain in the limbs and in the back of the head.

The patient passes little or no urine. He is generally in a stupor from the beginning, sometimes delirous, and even in a frenzy. Hearing, sight and touch are temporarily affected. Vomiting and diarrhœa are frequent.

His temperature may sink below normal, but in very serious cases it rises often very high.

Uremia sometimes lasts only a few days, but in

other cases it lasts weeks, months and even years. Most cases are curable by Nature Cure.

Treatment.—First of all a diet to reduce the formation of urea in the body; oatmeal-soup, fruit juices, buttermilk and bonnyclabber.

Secondly, stimulate the discharge of urine—give patient asparagus, parsley, watermelon (or tea of its seeds) and tea of juniper berries. Further, give the patient a kidney pack renewed every two hours, and twice a day a sitz bath of 95° F., and pour more and more boiling water into it until it reaches 110° to 113° F. Leave him in it an hour.

For constipation give patient enemas.

Frequent cold sponge baths, and every second day a bed steam-bath or foot steam, help much to expel the poison.

Rubbing and clapping of the kidneys help much to restore their normal functions.

VACCINATION.

Vaccination is a voluntary infectious disease caused by the physician's injection of pox poison into the human body, to make it, as they say, immune against smallpox.

It is hard to believe, however, that an *artificially poisoned body* should be better able to resist an epidemic than a quite or comparatively *healthy one.*

Further, no physician can prove to you that, nor how a human body grows immune against smallpox by poisoning it. The statistics they bring for it cannot be proved.

Many a very serious disease, as syphilis, scrofula and tuberculosis, has been inoculated into a formerly healthy body by it, and many deaths are caused by it, besides thousands being crippled and maimed for lifetime.

At the place of vaccination appears generally on the fourth day redness with a little knot in its middle, changing soon into a little pustula, in which there is pus, which later forms a scab, which falls off, leaving frequently a scar.

Often vaccination is accompanied by a high fever, convulsions, restless sleep, swelling of the arm and the lymphatics.

Many secondary diseases are caused by it. One of the most frequent is the very dangerous and fatal erysipelas.

Frequently vaccination causes inflammation of the nerves of the arm and total lasting lameness, although its bad effects often only appear slowly and after several years.

Many of these secondary diseases cause death.

Although quite a number of children seem to go through vaccination apparently unharmed, it ought to be abolished on account of the great harm it does in thousands and thousands of cases.

VOMITING.

Vomiting is not a disease in itself, but a symptom of many diseases, as:

Enlargement of the stomach,

Sores in stomach,
Catarrh of stomach,
Cancer of stomach,
Migraine,
Hysteria,
Cholera infantum,
Asiatic cholera,
Uremia,
Peritonitis,
Stricture of the bowels,
Liver trouble, etc.
Look for treatment of these diseases.

WARTS.

Hold them every hour a little while in cold water, and cover them with a pack during the night, or put onion juice on them, or freeze them till white, protecting the surroundings.

WATERBRASH.

Waterbrash (heartburn) is a symptom of a catarrh of the stomach. Look there for treatment.

WHOOPING-COUGH.

Whooping-cough is a disease of the bronchials.

Children from the seventh month to their seventh year are mostly affected by it.

It begins with slight changeable fever, loss of appetite and of cheerfulness, sleepiness, cough and sensitiveness to light.

Later on the cough grows worse, preceded by a whistling, gappy breathing. Heavy attacks of coughing last sometimes for ten or fifteen minutes and expel a tenacious mucus.

While coughing hard the child is a picture of misery, with a red or purple face, protruding eyes, as if suffocating. These attacks come more frequently during the night than in daytime, but between times the child is generally happy and bright.

After four to six weeks comes the more serious period. Although the attacks are rarer and not so long now, this is the period where the nursing of the child is of the greatest importance in order to prevent serious secondary diseases.

Separation as a prevention is often impossible and without the wanted effect. Therefore, give the well children every morning a cold sponge bath, and every evening a tub bath of 90° F. Let them gargle frequently during the day with lemon juice and water. Give them plenty of outdoor exercise and trunk and calf packs during the night. Also once or twice a week a vapor-bath or sweat.

We do not pretend that this will prevent whooping-cough in *all* cases, but it will certainly, if it should come, make it shorter and the coughing spells easier.

During the disease give the patient daily some vapor application; little children, foot steam; larger, not resisting children, a bed steam-bath. Do not give the latter to resisting children, as even the resistance will cause a coughing spell. Every sweat or vapor-bath ought to be followed by a tub bath of 85° or 90° F., ten to fifteen minutes.

During the night put patient into a trunk and calf packs, removed in the morning, and followed by a cold sponge bath or a tub bath, 90° F.

Let the child gargle frequently with water mixed with a little lemon juice. Do not say of a four or six-year-old child: "It cannot do it," but teach it. Children of two years can learn it.

Keep its bowels open with enemas, each evacuation followed by a remaining enema.

The diet must be mild. No meat, fish, eggs, wine or beer.

Take the yolk of an egg, beat it well, put in a tablespoonful of sugar and stir it into a hot lemonade. Give this warm, *not hot*, to the patient.

Fresh air is more needed by the patient than food; therefore he ought to sleep with wide-open windows, and take daily outdoor exercise; in summer let him remain all day outdoors.

Sun-baths and walking barefoot in summer make the whooping-cough of very short duration.

Whooping-cough treated thus with Nature's own healing factors is generally cured in four weeks, while with medical treatment it lasts often eighteen or twenty weeks.

WORMS.

Worms get into the system by what we eat, especially by meat.

Constipation alternately with diarrhœa, colic, flatulence, indigestion, itching in the nose, vomiting, a pale complexion with dark rings around the eyes, and restless sleep are general symptoms of worms.

To find out if a child has worms, let it drink some acid juice (lemon, cider, etc.), which drives out some of the worms.

Then give it for some time no meat, fish, etc., but only whole wheat bread, or graham bread, fruit, carrots, turnips and water.

Besides this give it every night an abdominal pack, and two enemas every day.

An occasional sweat and daily abdominal massage are very good.

WOUNDS.

Look up "POISONING."

YELLOW JAUNDICE.

This disease is caused by a mechanical obstacle preventing the flow of the bile from the biliary passages. Such an obstacle can be a diseased liver, or the biliary passages may be diseased themselves, or neighboring organs form an obstacle in time of sickness of such organs, as in stomach trouble, catarrh of the bowels, kidney trouble, womb trouble, etc.

The bile enters the blood, which causes the yellow discoloration of the skin, first appearing in the white of the eyes.

Later on the skin begins to itch, the urine grows greenish yellow or even reddish-brown. The fæces

12

are ash gray and very greasy, the tongue is coated, a bitter taste in the mouth, and the abdomen enlarged.

The liver is swollen, hard and painful to touch.

Sometimes it is accompanied by fever, delirium, headache and pain in the muscles.

The first improvement is shown in the fæces growing yellow, green or even brown again.

Treatment.—The diet has to be a very mild one—oatmeal, rice, barley, soft-boiled eggs, toast, fruit, lettuce, vegetables, lemonade, buttermilk, clabber and almond milk. Meat and all rich foods have to be avoided.

Give the patient daily two or three enemas of 70° F., and after the evacuation a remaining enema of a few spoonfuls of cold water.

The itching will be lessened and often it will entirely disappear by sponge baths of 72° F.

Further, give the patient two to four sitz baths daily of 90° F., half an hour each. These improve the action of the bowels, the secretion of bile, the appetite, lessen the headache and sleeplessness, and thus free the blood quickly from the bile, preventing an overloading of bile in the blood.

If there is a sharp pain in the liver give the patient a hot (110° F.) sitz bath, thirty minutes, and an hour before every meal a trunk pack, leaving it on till an hour after the meal.

Strong patients who have not a weak heart may take also an occasional vapor-bath.

Massage and physical culture exercises* and ''pick up pebbles,'' page 54, greatly hasten the recovery. So do air-baths and water treading.

*See Figures 3, 4, 5, 16.

ERRATA

PAGE 106.—Omit reference to Fig. 21 in foot note.

PAGES 160 AND 185.—Omit reference to Fig. 18 in foot note.

PAGE 189.—For Fig. 26 read Fig. 25, and for Fig. 25 read 26.

PAGE 191.—For Fig. 21 read Fig. 17.

A PACK consists of a wet part close to the body, and a larger dry part covering the wet. In Europe, where Nature Cure is spread everywhere, you can buy special material for packs—raw silk or coarse linen for the wet part, and thick flannel for the dry part.

The main purpose of a pack is to make the skin act and to draw the blood from other congested or inflamed parts. As soon as it grows warm the heat of the body produces a warm, agreeable moisture. This opens the pores, to which it draws at the same time the blood, and the impurities are pushed out into the damp cloth. As all diseases are caused more or less by an accumulation of poisons in the system, the main aim of Nature Cure is to take the poison out instead of increasing it with drugs, and for this purpose we give the packs; for if the skin acts well in the pack a great amount of poison comes out of millions of pores.

The skin is a very important organ, and on its

*See Figures 17 to 28.

PART III.

TREATMENTS EXPLAINED.

PACKS.*

A PACK consists of a wet part close to the body, and a larger dry part covering the wet. In Europe, where Nature Cure is spread everywhere, you can buy special material for packs—raw silk or coarse linen for the wet part, and thick flannel for the dry part.

The main purpose of a pack is to make the skin act and to draw the blood from other congested or inflamed parts. As soon as it grows warm the heat of the body produces a warm, agreeable moisture. This opens the pores, to which it draws at the same time the blood, and the impurities are pushed out into the damp cloth. As all diseases are caused more or less by an accumulation of poisons in the system, the main aim of Nature Cure is to take the poison out instead of increasing it with drugs, and for this purpose we give the packs; for if the skin acts well in the pack a great amount of poison comes out of millions of pores.

The skin is a very important organ, and on its

*See Figures 17 to 28.

action depends, in most diseases, the life and health of the patient. On account of this, whenever you or any of your dear ones feel sick in any way, do not wait for a disease to become pronounced, but give him directly a trunk pack and calf packs, which often prevent a serious disease from establishing itself, or make it at least less serious. In case the patient feels cold, however, let the packs be preceded by either a hot bath or by a short vapor application to the feet or to the whole body, for *no cold water application should ever be given to a cold body.*

Besides making the skin act and thus purifying the blood from its poisons the packs strengthen and soothe the nervous system. I have had many cases of very serious nervous disturbances where a single partial nerve pack soothed a very hysterical patient like a charm, and the patients often say they feel "newborn" after it.

1. The dry part of a pack must always be larger than the wet part, so that no cold air can reach the latter.

2. After every pack the packed part of the body should be washed with cool or cold water, or a bath of 90° F. given to the patient.

3. If you have never had a pack nor given one to anybody, try one yourself before giving one to anyone else; try it dry on the dressed patient in order to see if you can do it right.

4. Have everything ready before the patient undresses.

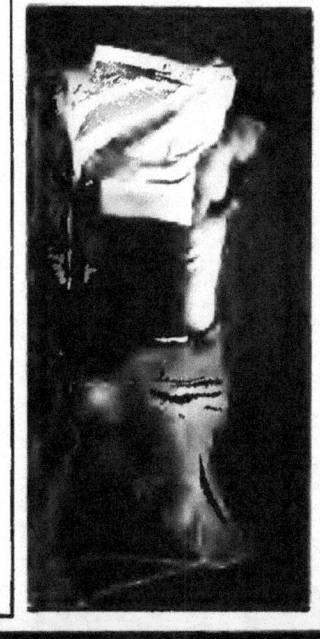

FIGURE 17. ABDOMINAL PACK

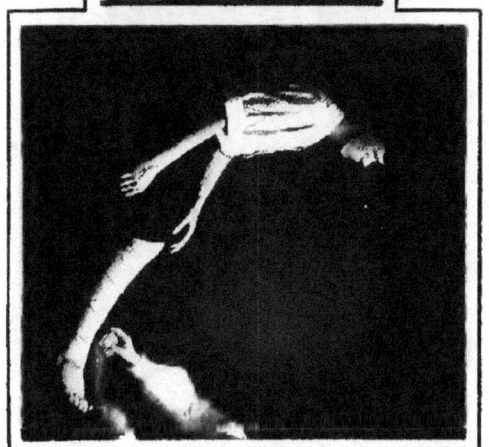

FIGURE 18. LEG PACK

5. If the body of the patient is warm, but his feet cold, give him first a hot foot bath or put directly a hot-water bag to his feet.

6. The pack should be applied quickly and very tightly pinned or tucked in, but not so tight as to prevent comfortable breathing.

7. With a whole pack the blanket should project beyond the sheet at least two or three inches at the neck and at the feet. If the sheet is longer turn it in. The size of the blanket for a grown person should be 2 x 2 yards.

8. If the patient is a very stout person and the blanket is not large enough to tuck it in well, take two, or pin the one at the edges where it pulls apart.

9. If after ten or fifteen minutes the feet do not grow warm in a pack put a hot-water bottle or heated brick to them.

10. During a dry pack (or sweat) keep a cold compress on patient's head all the time he is in it, renewed every three minutes.

11. In very high fever leave considerable water in the sheet, or take two sheets, but with a nerve pack wring it out very tight, especially the first time. If the patient this first time grows warm in it soon you may leave it a little wetter the next time, but if he has not grown comfortably warm after thirty minutes put hot bottles at his feet and near his legs, or (if he grows restless) take him out.

12. With very nervous patients we begin always with a partial nerve pack.

13. The average time for a fever pack is half an hour; in very high fever, less. In diseases without fever one and one-half hours or longer if the patient feels comfortable in it.

14. For very nervous patients, and patients who are not used to cold water, wring the pack out of water 90° or 95° F. in the beginning; later cooler by degrees.

15. After you have put on the pack, cover the patient with bedclothes according to the season, but on a dry pack (sweat), or bed steam-bath, put three or four quilts or even a feather bed, well tucked in, so that the perspiration may start quickly.

16. When in a dry pack the patient's upper lip grows moist, it is a sign that his body is perspiring.

17. Children generally cry considerably if you put them in a whole pack, because they cannot stand it to have their arms in; wherefore it is advisable to give them only three-quarter packs or other partial packs.

18. Many packs a person can put on himself, and with a little practice he grows quite proficient in it.

Abdominal Pack.—Put on the bed a two or three-fold piece of thick, dry flannel, two to five feet long, according to stoutness of patient, and 16 to 20 inches wide. On it put coarse, smooth linen or raw silk just as long, but four inches narrower, wrung out tightly in cold water.*

*See Figure 17.

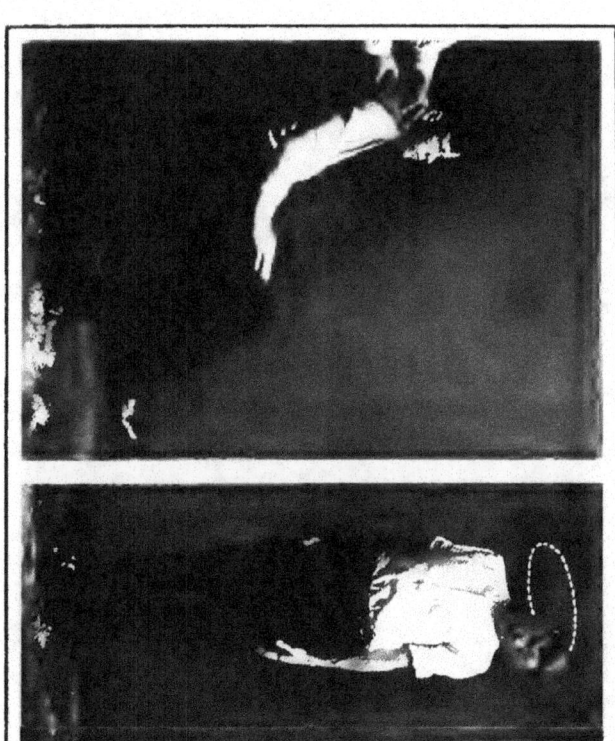

FIGURE 28   ARM PUSH.   FIGURE 6.   HEAD TURNING.

Let patient sit on the lower border of it, then lie down on it. Then wrap his abdomen tightly first in the wet parts and then in the dry flannel. Pin it very tightly with safety pins, especially at waist line of ladies, otherwise it would be loose there and feel chilly. Pull down patient's nightgown over it, and cover him with bedclothes according to the season.

Ankle Pack.—Take a strip of linen four to six feet long, three inches broad; wring it out in cold water and put it rather tightly alternately around the ankle and under the middle of the foot in form of an 8. Then take a strip of flannel four inches wide and three or four feet long and wrap it repeatedly over the wet part so that it covers the wet part one inch each side. Finally pin the end with a safety pin.*

Arm Pack.—Wrap rather tightly around the arm strips of wet linen, followed by dry strips of flannel well covering the wet parts. Fix a special strip of any material from top of shoulder around patient's neck to keep the upper part of the pack from slipping down.†

Calf Pack.—The calf of the leg is either done in the same way as the arm pack, or you may use for it the wet legs of white stockings covered with the dry legs of woolen ones.‡

*See Figure 18.
†See Figure 28.
‡See Figure 18,

Chest Pack. (Lung Pack).—Take a piece of soft, smooth linen, for instance a piece of an old table-cloth, about two yards long and about nine inches wide; wring it out in cold water; put it with its middle to the chest of the patient, and bring first one, then the other end underneath the arm, across the back over opposite shoulders, and join in front, over-lapping each other a little.*

Then take a piece of thick (or double) flannel, or part of a blanket, of same length but three or four inches wider, pulling it pretty tightly, and pin it at throat, at corner ends in front, at crossings at front and back of each arm, in back of neck and at the lower crossing of the back. Smooth and draw tight this latter part before pinning it with a safety pin.

Dry Pack (or sweat).—The dry pack is generally more effective when preceded by a hot bath. There-fore prepare a hot tub bath, 108° to 110° F., and have a basin with cold water and a rag near the bath tub for a compress for the head of the patient.

Then bring into a bedroom, near to the bathroom, many bed covers. Put on the mattress of the bed a thick pad or oilcloth covered with a blanket.

Let patient undress entirely and wrap himself in a large, thick blanket. Lead him to the bathroom and put him in the bath. Put directly the cold com-press on his head and renew it frequently. If the patient is lame, rheumatic or gouty, rub affected parts very gently towards the heart if the patient

*See Figures 22 and 23.

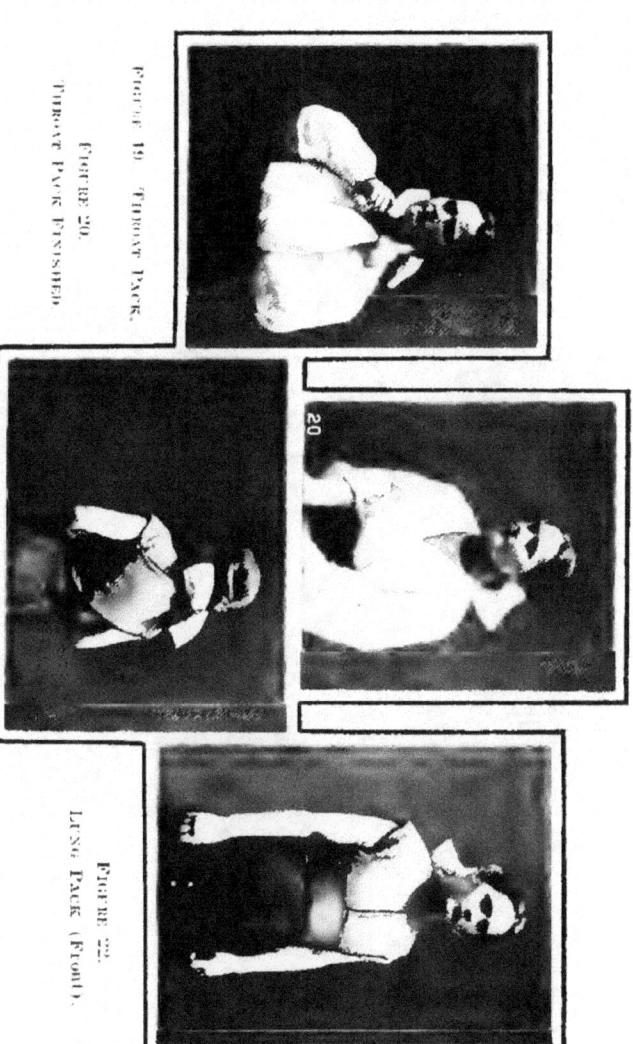

Figure 19. Throat Pack.

Figure 20.
Throat Pack Finished.

Figure 21. Lung Pack (Back).

Figure 22.
Lung Pack (Front).

is very nervous. But if he is not nervous rub deep while he is in the water.

Let more hot water run if patient can stand it. Leave him in ten minutes, after which bring him *slowly* into a sitting position, taking off the compress. Wrap him undried in the blanket and take him and the compress to bed. There put the compress directly on his forehead and wrap him up in the blanket, as explained under bed steam-bath; put many bed covers on him, well tucked in at the sides, and a hot-water bag to the feet, and renew the cold compress every two or three minutes.

If the upper lip of the patient grows moist after some time, it is a sign that he is perspiring. Leave him in the pack one hour unless he feels restless or oppressed, when you must take him out directly.

While he is in the pack prepare a 90° F. tub bath for him, in which you wash him off well after he comes out of the pack, and let him rest more or less according to the case.

The blanket he sweats in should be washed before it is used again, unless he has not perspired at all.

Little children are only wrapped up in the dry pack to underneath the arms, as they grow restless when they cannot have their arms out.

This sweat can be given to the weakest, even a dying person. It has given back to life and health many an almost dead person.

Eye Pack.—Take a tuft of absorbent cotton, dip it in cool 80° F. water, let the water run out until it only drips, put it on the patient's closed eye, cover with dry flannel and a tie over it, pinned at the back of the head.

Leave it on according to directions given in the case, and after its removal wash it with cool water or take an eye bath. This eye pack does good in any eye trouble. In highly inflamed eyes it should be renewed as soon as the heat is increasing again. Without inflammation it may stay on longer.

Foot Pack.—Never put a foot pack on cold feet. If they are cold warm them first, either by rubbing them or with a hot foot bath.

Take a pair of white cotton stockings which reach up to the patient's knees; wring them out in cold water and put them on patient's feet and lower legs. Then put over them one or two pairs of dry, thick, woolen stockings which cover well the wet ones, and in winter put him to bed. In summer time he may sit or walk about in them, provided they stay warm.

Kidney Pack.—A kidney pack is the same as an abdominal pack, only three inches higher up, and an extra damp cloth in the back at the waist line.

Leg Pack.—A leg pack is applied in the same way as an arm pack, as the picture shows.*

Partial Nerve Pack I.—Put a thick blanket on the bed, the upper border turned down four inches. Put on the middle of the upper part of the blanket, lengthwise from turned-in line downwards, a wet

*See Figure 18.

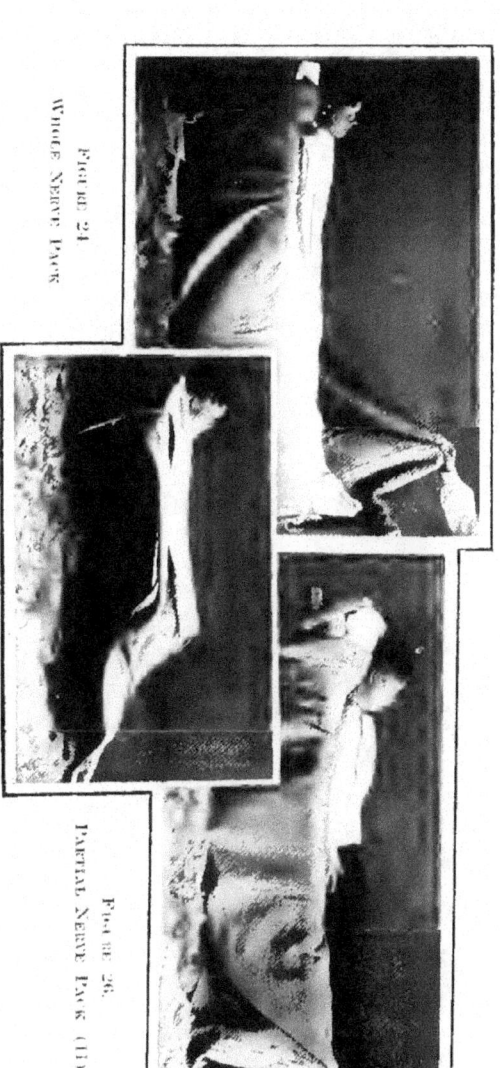

FIGURE 24.
WHOLE NERVE PACK

FIGURE 25. TRUNK BATH

FIGURE 26.
PARTIAL NERVE PACK (II.)

linen double strip, 6 x 18 inches. Let patient lie with bare back on the wet linen so that his spine rests on its middle.*

Then take in one of your hands one upper single corner of the blanket and draw it in a straight line with the middle front of patient's body. Put your other hand flat down on it with a gentle pressure underneath the chin of the patient, holding it there. The corner part in the other hand is drawn upwards over and behind the opposite shoulder of the patient and smoothly downwards. Then the lower part of that side of the blanket is wrapped tightly around the patient's body. Do the other side in the same way, and if the patient's feet are cold put a hot-water bag, or a heated brick, wrapped up, to his feet. Cover him with bedclothes and leave him in the bed according to directions given in the case.

When the time is up wash his back with cold water and dry it lightly, quickly and without much friction.

Partial Nerve Pack II.—This is the same as the preceding with the addition of another strip (same size) of linen put on the front of the body from the neck downwards.†

Three-Quarter Nerve Pack.—This is the same as a whole nerve pack, only that the wet sheet covers only three-quarters of the body, from the feet to the armpits.‡

*See Figure 26.
†See Figure 25.
‡See Figure 27.

In cold weather you may wrap the neck, arms and shoulders of the patient also in the blanket, while the wet sheet reaches only to the armpits.

Spinal Pack.—This is the same as Partial Nerve Pack I. But if it is given to a restless patient attach the wet part, covered with thick flannel, with strips around the waist, neck and shoulders in summer; in cooler weather by putting a vest of thick flannel underwear over it.

Tampon.—The tampon, as the picture shows, consists of absorbent cotton rolled up tightly, about 2½ inches long, and, according to width of the passage, as thick as a finger or thicker, with a clean thread around it knotted firmly. Dip it in cold water, squeeze it out, and insert it into the vagina (passage), letting the ends of the thread hang out, to draw it out by.*

It is, so to say, a pack of the vagina, and has a wonderfully curative effect in a number of female troubles, for instance, inflammations, catarrh of the womb, sores, infections, etc. If there are any sores or wounded places the tampon should be soaked in boiled and then cooled water mixed with lemon juice.

In dislocations of the womb a tampon is the best means to hold it in place, but the patient cannot insert it herself for this purpose.

It absorbs poisons, decomposed matter, cleanses and heals sores, cures leucorrhœa and inflammation, besides preventing dangerous infections if promptly used.

*See Figure 10.

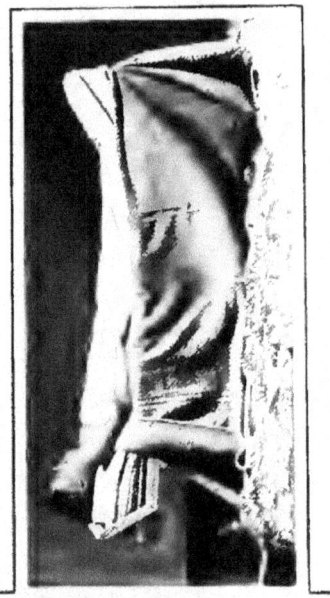

FIGURE 27. THREE-QUARTER NERVE FACE

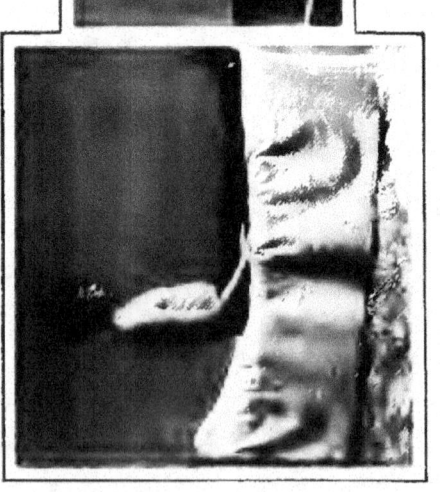

FIGURE 25. PARTIAL NERVE FACE (1).

Menstruation is not to prevent its use.

It is best inserted by making one end rather pointed. Part the lips with one hand and push the pointed end into the vagina till you feel it is high enough to stay with comfort. If you cannot make it stay, or if there is a dislocation of the womb, your physician should insert it, and he may be able to teach you how to do it yourself.

Do not leave it in longer than twelve hours.

Throat Pack.—Take a large linen handkerchief, double it lengthwise six or eightfold, according to length of the neck, wring it out in cold water and wrap it rather tightly around the neck, beginning in front, so that the throat is covered twice by the overlapping of the ends.*

Then put either a dry woolen stocking or a sleeve of thick woolen or cotton underwear around it, covering well the wet part, and pin it with a safety pin. After removing it, wash the neck with cold water.

Trunk Pack.—A trunk pack envelops the whole trunk of the body from the hip joints to the armpits; otherwise it is the same as an abdominal pack.†

Whole Nerve Pack.—Spread a thick, dry, large blanket on the bed. On it put a wet sheet and towel wrung out tightly in cool water 80°, or 90° F. to begin with. The upper end of the blanket is turned down four inches, so is the upper end of the sheet which touches at the double part of the blanket.‡

* See Figure 19.
† See Figure 21.
‡ See Figure 24.

Put the undressed patient on it so that he sits on lower line of the towel. Wrap this tightly around his abdomen. Then wrap the sheet well around him (between legs one side part); then the blanket as described in "dry pack." Cover him well with bed coverings, and if the feet are cold put a hot-water bag to them. Leave him in it forty to sixty minutes. If he warms up quickly you may make the sheet wetter next time. If he does not grow warm in thirty minutes take him out, and do not repeat it until he is improved, or take the water first 90° F.

With very nervous patients it is always better to begin with the Partial Nerve Pack I, then II, further the three-quarter pack, and then the whole nerve pack.

BATHS.

Alternate Sitz Bath.—Put two sitz baths (or washtubs) beside each other, in one hot (105° F.) water, in the other cool, 50° to 60° F., but only so much water that it will not overflow when patient sits in it. Stout persons fill it up considerably, consequently need little water. In a foot-tub in front of sitz baths have 108° to 110° F. water.

Put the patient alternately in the hot, then the cool tub, three times each, five minutes in the hot, one minute in the cold water. The foot tub goes from one to the other, as its water remains the same for the feet. Begin always with the hot and end always with the cool sitz bath. This is very successful in malarial fever.

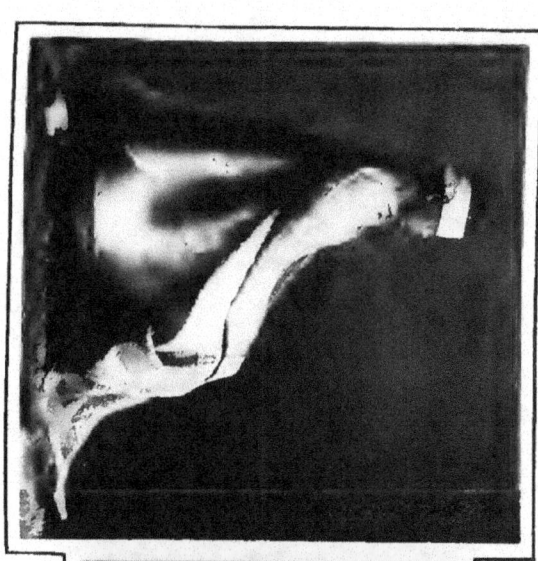

Figure 30. Vapor-Bath.

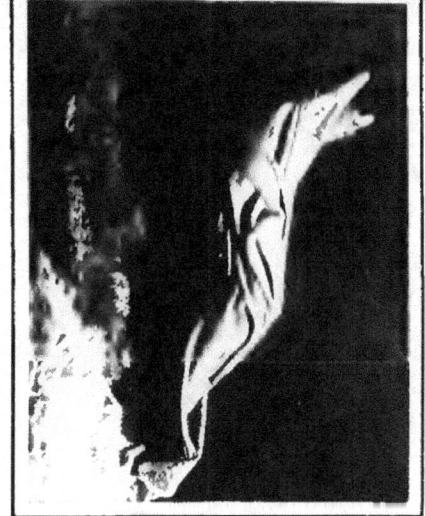

Figure 31. Sitz Bath.

Sitz Bath.—A sitz bath, as well as trunk bath, is of the greatest help in the treatment of diseases, especially in female trouble, against inflammations, pain, menstruation disorders, contractions, etc. They cleanse, heal, bring impurities to absorption, prevent puerperal fever, cause contraction of the womb after childbirth, quicken childbirth (hot), and in many other cases are of such great help that their effect often surpasses our greatest expectations.

A sitz bath has such a wonderful curative power in female trouble that we can almost regard it as a specific means for it. In painful menstruations, polypus, sores, catarrh of the womb, puerperal fever, inflammations of the vagina, the womb, ovaries, etc., it is unequaled in its healing, soothing and refreshing effects.*

If you have not a regular sitz bath, take a large washtub, put it against the wall and in front of it a foot tub with hot (108° to 112° F.) water. In sitz bath put only as much water as is needed to cover the navel of the patient when she (or he) sits in it, the degree according to case.

Put only as much water in it as is needed to fill it with the patient sitting down in it. Many people have a flood the first time because they put too much water in it; a stout patient fills it up so much.

After one bath has been taken, make a mark in the tub at the water line before dipping it out, so you will know exactly how much it takes for any future baths.

*See Figure 31.

18

Put before it a foot-tub or basin with hotter water for the feet, or a hot-water bag to rest the feet on.

The temperature of the water and the length of time are according to the case and should be looked up under the proper ailment.

In cold weather spread a blanket over the patient, pinning it behind the back of tub with a safety pin.

Alternate Foot Bath.—This is on the same order as the alternate sitz bath, with the only difference that no other part of the body but the feet are bathed.

It is best taken on a chair before which either two buckets or foot tubs with hot and cool water stand, and the feet put alternately into them.

They are very useful in gout, rheumatism in feet, bunions, sciatica, swollen feet, chilblains, weak feet (flat feet), especially when followed by massage. Begin with the hot water and end with the cold.

Bed Steam Bath.—Heat five earthen jars or bottles; fill them with boiling water and keep them hot on the stove in a pan with hot water. Then put on a bed two thick blankets, on which you put a double strip of linen or raw silk wrung out in cold water, 24 inches wide and long enough to go well around the trunk of the patient's body.

After you have put the patient on it, wrap it well around the trunk of his body from hips to armpits. Then wrap cold, wet cloths also around the calves of his legs. Then wrap the uppermost blanket well around him, put the hot jars or bottles (wrapped in

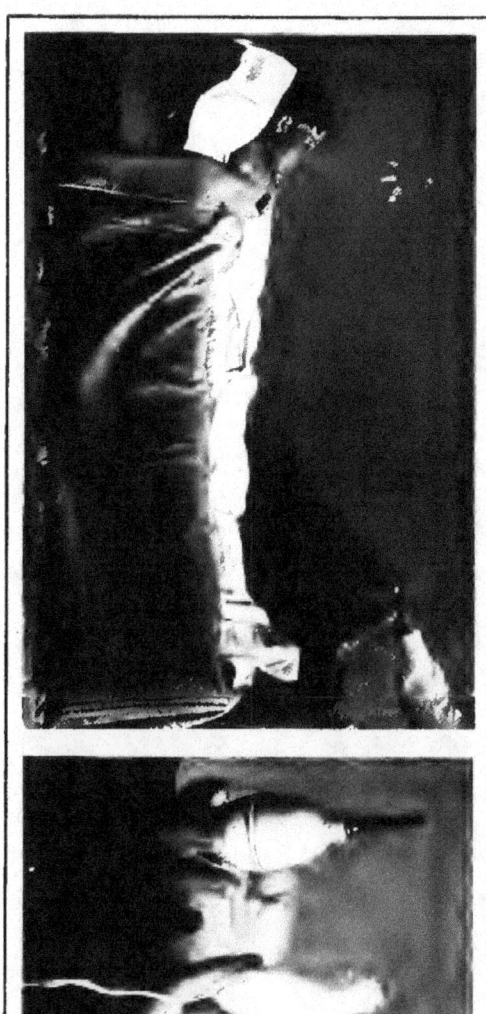

FIGURE 29   BED STEAM-BATH.

FIGURE 10
INFANT SYRINGE AND TAMPON.

wet rags), one across his feet, one against each calf of leg, and one against each side of the trunk of his body. Instead of the hot bottles you can take hot ears of corn, boiled with the husks. Then wrap all into the lower blanket, especially tight around the neck. Put many bedclothes over him, and a pillow between the bedstead and the bottle at feet, all tucked in well, and a cold, wet cloth on his forehead, renewed every three minutes. Leave him in it one to two hours, but not longer than he feels comfortable in it. Then take him out and give him a warm 90° F. bath, five to eight minutes, or a cold sponge bath. This is a milder form of vapor-bath than the one in the cabinet. (See Figure 29.)

Eye Bath.—Take an eye glass (sold in drug stores), fill it to the brim with 75° F. water, press the eye gently into it and bend the head back. Hold it there from three to five minutes, then do the same with the other eye. Repeat these eye baths four to six times a day.

Face Bath.—Put cold water into a wash-basin, breathe deep and put your face into it and out for about a minute. For breathing intervals raise either the face out of the water for a moment or only the mouth above the surface of the water. It improves the complexion wonderfully.

Head Bath.—Put a wash-bowl with 70° to 90° F. water on the floor. Before it put some pillows or a folded quilt to nearly the height of the basin. Then lie on the quilt and put the back of your head into the water, turning it now and then a little sideways.

Take it from eight to twelve minutes, according to feeling and case.

It is very good for any skin diseases of the head, rheumatism, gout, ear and eye troubles, pain in eyes and dandruff.

Half Bath.—For certain ailments we prefer a half bath to a full tub bath.

For a grown person put only eight inches of water (for children less) into the bathtub, so that when patient lies down it will not cover the heart.

Put one of your arms on slanting head part of the tub, the hand with outspread fingers downwards; rest the patient's head on this arm, while with the other hand you gently and rhythmically wave the water over the chest of the patient for ten or twelve minutes.

Then put the patient into a sitting position, and pour cooler or cold water, according to directions in the case, on the upper back of the patient.

This bath has a wonderful effect on the nerves and heart, and is always used in pneumonia, typhoid fever and many other diseases with great success.

Mouth Bath.—Mouth baths are used with great success for a sore throat, inflammation, catarrh, nervous affections, hoarseness, all diseases of the vocal chords and the ears.

They refresh, cleanse, heal, dissolve and draw out impurities, soothe the pain, and cause a great excretion of mucus.

They are best taken in a lying position. Take of cold water (if your teeth can stand it) a swallow in your mouth, close the lips, but separate the teeth so that the water flows back as much as possible; hold it there till it grows warm and spit it out.

Repeat.

Do this for fifteen or twenty minutes at a time, and in serious troubles every hour in the day. If there are sores in the throat add a little lemon juice to the water.

In cases where the nose is affected too, draw cold or cool water up the nostrils, but not with too much force, as that would cause a headache.

Sand Bath.—As a sand bath consists of bathing or lying in hot sand, the seashore or bank of a river are, on a summer day, the most convenient places for it. It may also be taken in your own yard.

Make a long hole in the hot sand, according to size of patient's body, slanting at head part, throwing the dug-out sand all around, but not on a heap, so that the sun heats it quickly.

After the sand in the hole is *well* heated put the undressed patient into the hole and cover him up to his chin with the surrounding *upper* hot sand. Shade his eyes with a chair, an umbrella, or a newspaper, and leave him in it for an hour or longer if he feels comfortable and hot in it. Then take him out and wash him off, either in the near ocean, or river, or tub, according to place and conveniences.

This bath has a wonderful effect in rheumatism,

gout, paralysis, double joints (rachitis), ṣkin diseases and scrofula, especially so when followed by massage and gymnastics of the ailing parts.

Spinal Patting.—Take hold of the middle of a laundry-folded towel, dip one end of it in cold water and squeeze a little out of it, and pat (or slap) gently up and down the spine of patient. Do not rub to dry the spine, but hold a dry towel against it for a few seconds.

Sponge Bath.—For most people it is advisable to take a sponge bath in a warm room in winter time, and river baths in summer.

Rub all parts of your body with cold or cool water, dry *lightly,* limbs upwards, and dress.

Very delicate persons are not dried at all, but go back into the warm bed for ten minutes or so until quite dry.

Chilly persons can begin with a dry rub of a towel, which they dampen every day a little more; or begin with tepid water.

Too much friction irritates and finally lames the nerves of the skin.

Trunk Bath.—This bath is given in the same way as a sitz bath, only the effect is for some organs different, as the water covers more of them than in a sitz bath.*

If the legs of the patient are not long enough to be comfortable in a foot-tub before it, put them with

*See Figure 21.

a hot-water bag on a stool. If no trunk bathtub is available it can be taken in an ordinary bathtub; foot-tub raised, with heavy weight in it to keep it from floating. These baths are especially good for acute and chronic diseases of most organic troubles.

Vapor - Bath.—If you have no vapor cabinet or frame do the following: Take an old chair with an open (cane, etc.) seat, put in the middle underneath it a little low stove, with a pretty deep pan of boiling water on it.*

Take four layers of a double-sheeted newspaper, or other paper, of which you put five sheets on the seat, and let three hang down in front of the chair.

Put the undressed patient on the chair, and pin three to four thick blankets or an old quilt around him up to his neck.

Around his head, to cool his forehead, pin a narrow folded towel of which the middle part is wrung out of cold water.

Give him at the beginning and a few minutes later a glass of water to drink, if he likes it.

Renew the head compress every three minutes.

When the patient's upper lip grows damp, it is a sign that his body is perspiring.

Leave him in it for fifteen to twenty-five minutes if he can stand it, longer if the vapor does not come freely from the water.

When you take him out give him either a half bath of 90° F. for five or eight minutes, or a cold sponge bath.

*See Figure 30.

Weak persons have to rest after it.

The vapor-bath must not be given to patients with very serious organic lung or heart trouble without the advice of a physician. Take a bed steam bath.

The vapor-bath is the "Pearl of Nature Cure," because it, more than any other means of cure, removes the deadly poisons, the cause of all diseases, out of the system. This shows most evidently in cases of blood poisoning, for as soon as the skin acts freely, pushing out the poison by perspiration, the patient is saved.

Enema.—Put water of temperature prescribed into a fountain syringe, hang it up on the wall, lie or kneel down, and after having let the air out of the tube of the syringe insert the greased point into the rectum. Then open the clasp to let the water flow. Close the clasp a moment if the water runs so freely as to cause pain, and open again to let flow more.

When enough is injected remain in the same position for fifteen or twenty minutes if possible before going to the toilet.

Foot Steam.—Before a high chair put a foot-tub with boiling water. On top of the foot-tub put two or three narrow sticks to rest your feet upon. Wrap a blanket around yourself, the chair and foot-tub.

When the vapor decreases let somebody pour more boiling water into it.

Do this for thirty to sixty minutes, then take either a cold sponge bath or a tub bath of 90° F.

For little children no sticks are needed on the

tub, as their feet hang over it and will not touch the water.

A foot steam is used in all cases where we want to draw the blood from other parts of the body downwards.

Fomentation or Vapor Compress.—In a pot of boiling water put a towel folded to the size the compress is to be. Take it out with a stick or large spoon, put it on a dry towel with which you wring it out in order not to burn your hands, put compress quickly between thick, dry flannels and place it on the patient. If very hot, and the patient is very sensitive to heat, put another thick layer of flannel underneath it. Cover with bedclothes and renew by another when cooling off.

Take a double set of towels and flannels, so that the one is always ready before you take the other one off.

These fomentations are very effective with suppuration, for instance, in the lungs (with pleuritis) or in the lymphatic glands at the neck. They draw the pus to the surface, and in most cases it bursts through the skin under the vapor compress, thus making an operation unnecessary.

Head Vapor.—Put on a table or chair a basin with boiling water, bend over it with a large towel or cloth over your head to keep the steam together. If there is no flame under the basin to keep the water boiling it has to be renewed if the vapor stops before the time is up. Length of time according to directions. After it wash off the face with cool or cold water and also gargle with cool water.

This head vapor relieves neuralgic pains in the head very promptly.

Pour or Gush.—Take a large sprinkler without the spray part, or a large pitcher, fill it with cold or tepid water as prescribed, and pour it on the patient in an easy even stream. For:

A back-pour on upper back.

A chest-pour on upper chest and shoulders.

A knee-pour on the knees alternately.

A neck-pour on back of the neck.

A head-pour on top of the head.

An arm-pour on upper arms alternately.

A stomach-pour on stomach.

A liver-pour on the liver (right lower ribs).

An abdominal-pour on abdomen around the navel—right side up, left side down.

Potato Poultice.—The very best poultice is a potato poultice, because it keeps the heat very long, and it is clean and easily handled.

Fill two square white bags half full of peeled potatoes, and sew them up. Then put them into boiling water and cook till the potatoes are done. Then crush them well in one, and put the poultice on as hot as the patient can stand it. Then crush the other well, and put it on when the first is cooling, which goes back into the boiling water, and so on alternately, according to directions given in case.

Remaining Enema.—Fill a baby syringe full of cold water. To make sure it is not party filled with air, squeeze it three or four times, and, pressing it, hold point in the water, relax the pressure, hold it up and squeeze it again. There is no more air in it if, when squeezing, the water comes out directly.*

Then insert it into the rectum, squeeze, hold a few seconds and draw out *while squeezing;* otherwise the water flows back into it.

The water is absorbed by the rectum and moistens, refreshes and strengthens it and all its surroundings.

It is given after every movement of the bowels and also between times for chronic constipation, croup, in most acute diseases, local inflammations of abdominal parts, etc.

Self Massage.—Self massage of the abdomen is performed by locking the hands, pressing them on the abdomen, and going around and around for ten minutes or more, left side down, right side up.

Massage of the Head.—Put the points of all your fingers apart above forehead and rub them gently backwards over the scalp of the head. Ten minutes every morning and evening will make the hair grow wonderfully, if roots are not destroyed.

Massage of the Stomach.—Put the three middle fingers of your right hand underneath your breast bone, and run them with as deep a pressure as you

*See Figure 10.

can stand below the right ribs; then do the same with left hand on the left side, and so alternately for eight or ten minutes every morning and evening.*

This massage, with *very long* masticating of your food, cures the most obstinate indigestion and catarrh of the stomach.

Massage of the Throat.—Hold your four fingers together and thumb apart, put thus the hands alternately to your neck, rubbing downwards along the throat. Do not press on the windpipe nor run fingers and thumb together when you come down, for by it all benefit would be lost and harm done.†

Inhaling Vapor.—Put a little gas stove or oil stove on the floor. On it put a tea kettle with its spout corked up and boiling water in it. Remove its lid and put on the opening a tube made of stiff paper 15 to 18 inches high. Sit on a chair before it and inhale the vapor for fifteen or twenty minutes.

To prevent the wind from blowing the vapor away, hang a large towel over your head and the back of a chair in front of you, on the other side of the stove.

After the inhalation gargle with tepid water or with water and lemon juice.

If your feet are cold, put them into a tub with hot water while you inhale the vapor.

Inhaling vapor is very good for all kinds of throat trouble, deafness from catarrh, tonsillitis, hoarseness, sore throat, etc.

*See Figure 2.
†See Figure 1.

PART IV.

HYGIENIC COOKING.

Only a well-nourished body can be healthy and strong, and in order to be well fed we ought to know what and how to eat, and how to prepare it.

Everyone knows that we need for the building up of the body certain quantities of albumen, fat, etc.; but too little attention is paid to the necessary minerals, and it is of the greatest importance for the body to have the proper amount of these as well.

Why are so many sedentary people anæmic? Because their diet consists mostly of meats, grains and the legumes, which are particularly poor in soda and lime. If to this diet a certain amount of vegetables and fruits were added, their blood and bones would grow healthier. For many it is sufficient to acquire a taste for vegetables, and even when they do have them they are in most cases unwholesome, being unhygienically prepared, so that they are robbed of most of their hygienic properties. In order to retain within the vegetables these properties they should never be washed in hot water, nor should the water in which they are cooked be poured off, for it contains in solution the strength-giving minerals of the vegetable. Therefore vegetables should be cooked in a very little water or steamed.

Besides that, few people know how to eat. If most people ailing from stomach trouble would only masticate their food every bite five times as long as they have been doing they would soon see a great change.

Naehrsalz.—Dr. Lahmann, of Germany, seeing the necessity of adding to certain vegetables the mineral salts they lack, discovered, after long and various experiments, a process by which to make a preparation from the mineral substances of plants, which he appropriately calls "Naehrsalz," or nutritious extract. It is particularly useful in our diet, since we can with it make many of our dishes more wholesome and digestible. We add it to meats and to those vegetables which do not contain a sufficient amount of the necessary minerals. Naehrsalz not only aids digestion, but improves the flavor of the food. It is to be added to a dish only shortly before serving it, and for a dishful of vegetables, naehrsalz the size of a pea only is needed.

Lahmann's Cocoa we have found to be the best and purest cocoa. It is made from the finest selected cocoa beans, is chemically free from grease and contains naehrsalz, which improves its flavor and makes it more easily digested.

The naehrsalz, the cocoa, chocolate and the vegetable milk of Dr. Lahmann can be had at the store of B. Lust, 124 East Fifty-ninth street, New York City.

Mr. B. Lust is one of the first naturopaths in the United States, and editor of one of the best monthly health magazines, published in English and German.

Konut we use in our kitchen for frying, shortening, etc. It is a pure vegetable fat, and is more easily digested than any animal fat. Finley Acker Co., of Philadelphia, Pa., sell it. Ask for the freshest.

Grape Juice is the pure juice of the grape, entirely free from alcohol and one of the most wholesome and nourishing beverages. We use it for our patients, since we never under any circumstances give alcoholic drinks.

Lemon Spice is made thus: Grate off the yellow part of lemon peel, mix it up with a good deal of granulated sugar and put it in a glass jar. It keeps for years when tightly closed. More peel may be added at any time. It is to be used only in small quantities, as spices of all kinds make the blood impure. We therefore use very little even of salt.

Breadsticks are especially to be recommended to give to a teething baby, in disorders of digestion, to people who "swallow their food;" they are always a great help when fresh bread is not available, and on picnics, camping, etc. They keep ever so long in a tin box.

Gruenkorn is rye harvested before growing mealy. It can be bought in most delicatessen stores of large cities. It is very wholesome, tasty and nourishing.

We have tried to explain German dishes as clearly as possible, and hope we have succeeded in doing so.

DRY DIET.

Schroth Cure.—The dry diet cure is also called "Schroth Cure," because Dr. Schroth invented it and made wonderful cures with it.

It consists of a diet reduced in fluids and mainly nothing but cereals, toast and some vegetables. The purpose of the dry diet is to condense the fluids in the patient's body so that they can do better work. The organs get a rest, and the power of the body is reawakened and strengthened.

In the absence of superfluous water the dormant poisons in our system dissolve and are expelled more readily by the natural channels, which is so evidently shown in the deep color (and often thick sediment) in the urine.

A strictly severe dry diet can only be entered upon with a knowing person to advise you. But a moderately dry diet can be followed for a few weeks by a strong person without any harm. It consists of the following three scanty meals every day:

1. Breakfast.—A cup of almond milk, oatmeal, toast.

2. Dinner.—Rice, barley or oatmeal, vegetables, toast.

3. Supper.—Fruit, toast, a cup of almond milk.

Further, every day either a whole or three-fourth nerve pack for two to four hours, or for four days in the week, and three days in the week a bed steam-bath.

Much outdoor exercise and breathing exercises should be taken.

Feel your pulse every day, morning and evening, and if it should go below 58, drink some unfermented grape juice, or fresh, pure water.

Watch your urine, and when it grows to a darker color and shows a sediment it is a sign of an effectual cure.

When you feel badly with it in any way, stop for a time and change to a greater variety in diet, but not suddenly to a banquet.

Weak persons ought not to undertake it unadvised.

It is used with dropsical swellings, cysts, hydrophobia, various organic troubles, etc.

Daily general massage makes it more effective.

MILD DIET.

"Under a mild diet" we understand to be a diet free from alcoholic drinks, coffee, tea, meat, sweets, rich or highly seasoned food, cake, etc., consisting of cereals, milk, almond milk, apple sauce, light vegetables and toast.

14

MENUS.

BREAKFASTS.

First Day:

Fresh fruit.
Health.
Boiled eggs and lettuce.
Breadsticks.
Muffins.
Honey.
Any cereal coffee or Dr. Lahmann's cocoa.

Second Day:

Cooked fruit.
Wheat hearts with sugar and cream.
Scrambled eggs and radishes.
Toast.
Honey.
Same drinks as first day.

Third Day:

Fresh fruit.
Grits with sugar and cream.
Poached eggs and watercress.
Corn bread and honey.
The same drinks as first day.

Fourth Day:

Cooked fruit.
Health.
Corn pancakes or breadsticks.
Maple syrup.
The same drinks.

Fifth Day:

Fresh fruit.
Wheat hearts.
Eggs on toast.
Honey.
The same drinks.

Sixth Day:

Cooked fruit.
Cream of wheat.
Corn muffins.
Soft boiled eggs and lettuce.
Honey.
The same drinks.

Seventh Day:

Fresh fruit.
Instantaneous tapioca.
Breadsticks.
Scrambled eggs and celery.
Honey.
The same drinks.

DINNERS.

JANUARY—FEBRUARY—MARCH.

January 1st:

Fresh fruit. Barley soup.
Cauliflower, baked.
Fried chicken.
Red cabbage with apples.
Mashed potatoes.
Celery salad.
Pueckler ice cream.
Bread and butter.
Cranberry sauce—nuts.

January 2d:

Fresh fruit.
Chestnuts.
Green beans.
Veal chops.
Irish and sweet potatoes.
Lettuce.
Tapioca pudding.
Breadsticks.

January 3d:

Stewed fruit.
Cabbage.
Dried peas with fried onions
(gravy).
Mutton roast.
Chestnuts.
Baked sweet potatoes.
Celery.
Chocolate cream.
Bread and butter.

January 4th:

Fresh fruit.
White beans.
Spinach with hard-boiled eggs.
Boiled fish.
Potato dumplings with butter
gravy.
Lettuce.
Bread and butter.
Breadsticks.
Nuts and raisins.

January 5th:

Stewed peaches.
Corn.
Green peas.
Veal roast.
Irish and sweet
potatoes.
Tomatoes, baked.
Pecan pudding.
Bread and butter.

January 6th:

Fresh fruit.
Asparagus.
Lettuce.
Cold meat jelly.
Potato salad.
Celery.
Apple pudding.
Bread and butter.
Nuts and raisins.

January 7th:

Cooked prunes.
Vegetable soup.
Chestnuts.
Stewed onions.
Smoked ox tongue.
Potato pancakes.
Mashed potatoes.
Lemon cream.
Breadsticks.

These menus may be repeated unchanged during the three winter months, or varied according to circumstances and taste.

APRIL—MAY—JUNE.

April 1st:

Stewed fruit.
Gruenkorn slices.
Spinach with hard-boiled eggs.
Chicken.
Fried Irish potatoes.
Sliced tomatoes.
Chocolate pudding.
Bread and butter.
Nuts.

April 2d:

Strawberries.
Green peas.
Vegetarian ragout.
Mutton chops.
Artificial chestnuts.
Lettuce.
Rice pudding.
Breadsticks.
Nuts.

April 3d:

Prune dumplings.
Carrots.
Rice-dish.
Veal roast.
Mashed Irish potatoes.
Baked sweet potatoes.
Lettuce.
Tutti-frutti.
Breadsticks.

April 4th:

Stewed fruit.
Vegetable slices.
Macaroni dish.
Beef roast.
Potato dumplings.
Sweet potatoes.
Celery salad.
Charlotte russe.
Bread and butter.

April 5th:

Strawberries.
Pea soup.
Cabbage, apples.
Corn with okra.
Onions.
Boiled fish.
Fried potatoes.
Red flammery.
Breadsticks.

April 6th:

Fresh fruits, nuts.
Spinach with eggs.
Chestnuts.
Stewed chicken.
Gruenkorn.
Sweet potatoes.
Irish potatoes.
Bread and butter.

April 7th:

Cooked fruit.
Dried peas with
  fried onions.
Asparagus.
Corn dumplings.
Irish potatoes.
Celery.
Orange cream.
Bread and butter.
Nuts.

Repeat.

JULY—AUGUST—SEPTEMBER.

July 1st:

Fresh fruit.
Green beans.
Rice with apples.
Mutton roast.
Mashed Irish potatoes.
Bean salad.
Lemon jelly.
Breadsticks.

July 2d:

Stewed fruit and raisins.
Cucumbers.
Pea slices.
Veal chops.
Tomato dish.
Potatoes.
Vanilla pudding.
Bread and butter.

July 3d:

Fresh fruit.
Cabbage.
Macaroni.
Fried chicken.
Potato pancakes.
Lettuce.
Chocolate pudding.
Bread and butter.

July 4th:

Stewed fruit.
Bean soup.
Egg plant.
Mushrooms.
Sauerkraut.
Mutton chops.
Mashed potatoes.
Celery.
Flammery.
Bread and butter.

July 5th:

Fresh fruit.
Vegetable ragout.
Green beans.
Tomatoes.
Steak.
Sour potatoes.
Fruit compote.
Breadsticks.

July 6th:

Fresh fruit.
Rice dish.
Pea slices.
Cauliflower.
Boiled fish.
Potato dumplings.
Almond pudding
    with fruit juice.
Bread and butter.

July 7th:

Cherry dumplings.
Noodles.
Spinach with eggs.
Mushrooms.
Veal chops.
Potato balls.
Sliced tomatoes.
Pueckler ice cream.
Breadsticks.

Repeat.

OCTOBER—NOVEMBER—DECEMBER.

October 1st:

Fresh fruit.
German kale.
Sweet corn.
Sliced tomatoes.
Boiled fish.
Mashed potatoes.
Breadsticks.
Nuts.

October 2d:

Apple dumplings.
Rice soup with tomatoes.
Spinach with sliced eggs.
Stewed chestnuts.
Potatoes with apples.
Fried chicken.
Celery.
Tutti-frutti.
Bread and butter.

October 3d:

Fresh fruit.
Green peas.
Turnip greens.
Stewed tomatoes.
Rabbit stew.
Bread pudding.
Bread and butter.

October 4th:

Apple sauce with canned peaches.
Kohlrabi.
Oyster plant.
Sliced Irish potatoes, fried.
Lettuce.
Stewed chicken.
Rice pudding.
Breadsticks.
Nuts and raisins.

October 5th:

Fresh fruit.
Chestnuts.
Green peas.
Rice.
Irish and sweet potatoes.
Sliced tomatoes.
Veal chops.
Chocolate pudding.
Bread and butter.
Nuts.

October 6th:

Canned peaches.
Spinach with eggs.
Corn.
Beet salad.
Celery.
Stewed chicken.
Mashed potatoes.
Rice pudding.
Breadsticks.

October 7th:

Rhubarb compote.
Green beans and corn.
Cabbage with apples.
Turkey.
Irish potatoes.
Chocolate cream.
Bread and butter.
Nuts.

Repeat.

COOKING RECIPES.

HOT SOUPS.

In using yolks of eggs in soups care must be taken that they do not harden in lumps in the soup. In order to avoid this, first beat them well and stir into them a few tablespoonfuls of the soup and beat together until thoroughly mixed and smooth; then pour this into the soup.

VEGETABLE SOUP STOCK.

One onion, 2 potatoes, 1 stick of celery, 2 carrots, 1 slice of egg plant, 1 slice of squash, a handful of black-eyed peas (fresh or dried), a little parsley, a handful of asparagus and two ounces of butter.

After having washed the vegetables, cut all into pieces and stew in the heated butter for awhile; then add a little boiling water and boil until done, after which stir all through a sieve. This vegetable stock is used for a number of soups.

VEGETABLE SOUP.

Green peas, snap beans, carrots, cauliflower, celery, onion, parsley, kohlrabi, potatoes, squash, black-eyed peas (in shell).

Put butter in a pot on the fire; when heated stir into it one-half tablespoonful of flour until it is a dark yellow; pour boiling water into it, a little salt and all or most of the above vegetables (which have been washed and cut) and boil until done. Finally, just before serving, add the yolks of three eggs.

SPLIT PEA SOUP.

Put 4 ounces of split peas in cold water and boil until done, and then strain them through a sieve. Meanwhile fry a spoonful of fine cut onions in 1½ ounces of butter and add to it the necessary amount of soup vegetables, the strained peas and a little salt; boil awhile. Serve with dices of toast.

The same soup may be made with black-eyed peas and green peas.

PEA SOUP.

One pint of green peas (or French peas). Boil with 3 ounces of butter over a moderate fire; sprinkle 1½ or 2 tablespoonfuls of flour over it, add the necessary amount of water, a little salt and vegetable stock and boil until done. Add the yolks of 2 eggs and serve over slices of toast.

WHITE BEAN SOUP.

One pound of white beans, 1½ ounces of butter, 1¾ ounces of flour, salt, vegetable stock.

Wash the beans and put them in rain water on a moderate fire; boil until done and then stir through a hair sieve. Brown the flour, add the beans, salt and vegetable stock. If too thick, add a little warm water. Boil one-half hour longer, and just before serving drop in toasted bread cut in squares or dice.

ASPARAGUS SOUP.

Peel 1 pound of cut and washed asparagus and boil in salted water or beef soup till done. Melt 3 ounces of butter in a pan, 2 tablespoonfuls of flour; stir awhile and then add the water of the asparagus. Before serving beat the yolks of 2 or 3 eggs in the tureen. Add 8 or 10 spoonfuls of the soup, being careful to beat continually the yolks to prevent hardening. Then add the rest of the soup and strew over it fine chopped parsley.

CAULIFLOWER SOUP.

This soup is made like asparagus soup, except that before serving lemon juice, to taste, may be added.

GRUENKORN SOUP.

Boil 3 or 4 ounces of gruenkorn in a little water slowly for four or five hours, now and then adding a little more water. Stir through a fine sieve; let it come to a boil again, adding salt, vegetable stock and 1½ ounces of butter. If the soup is too thin, thicken with a teaspoonful of flour dissolved in milk and pour it into the soup, stirring the while. Before serving, add the yolk of one egg and farina dumplings.

SPINACH SOUP.

Clean and wash ½ peck of spinach; boil in a little water; put 1½ ounces of butter in a pot, add the spinach and boil for awhile, adding a little salt, 2 tablespoonfuls of corn-starch and as much water as is needed. Serve with little crackers.

A soup may be made in the same way of squash.

TOMATO SOUP.

Wash and boil 2 pounds of tomatoes; when done stir through a hair sieve; beat ¼ pound of butter mixed with 2 tablespoonfuls of corn-starch and stir into tomato stock, together with a little salt, naehrsalz size of a pea (see page 206). Add the necessary amount of water and some parsley chopped fine. After boiling 20 minutes longer, take from the fire, and before serving pour into it one-half pint of cider.

PEANUT SOUP.

Peel and grate 4 ounces of peanuts; put 1 quart of buttermilk on a moderate fire; stir constantly until it comes to a boil, then pour it over the grated peanuts. Add a little salt, sugar and ½ tablespoonful of meal and let it boil 20 minutes, stirring all the while. Take from the fire and add the yolks of 2 eggs.

POTATO SOUP.

Cut into pieces 1½ pounds of peeled and washed potatoes; boil them in salted water till done and then put with the same water through a sieve. Meanwhile fry a tablespoonful of onions cut fine and 1 tablespoonful of flour to a light brown in 2 ounces of butter; pour cold water to it; add them and vegetable stock to the potatoes.

LENTIL SOUP.

Soak 1 pound of lentils over night in rain water; next morning put them over a moderate fire in the same water in which they were soaked, and cook till thoroughly done. If needed, add cold rain water now and then; put through a hair sieve; brown one tablespoonful of flour and one-half fine chopped onion in 2 ounces of butter and stir into the soup. Salt to taste.

MUSHROOM SOUP.

Wash 1 pound of mixed mushrooms; chop them, not fine; add 3 ounces of butter, ½ onion, a little fine chopped parsley. Stew slowly awhile; add the necessary amount of water and boil till done. Brown a little flour in butter, add it to the soup and stir into it, just before serving, the yolks of 2 eggs.

A very good soup for convalescents.

WHITE CABBAGE SOUP.

Shave 1 pound of white cabbage fine; cook till well done; add to it a little salt, 1 tablespoonful of corn-starch, dissolved in cold water, 2 tablespoonfuls of fresh butter, 1 egg, one-half bottle of cider, and serve with snowflake crackers or breadsticks.

PRUNE SOUP.

Wash prunes (fresh or dried) in cold water and cook in a little cold water over a moderate fire till done; put them through a sieve and sweeten to taste. In another pot put about 1 quart of milk and mix with it 2 or 3 tablespoonfuls of corn-starch and bring it to a boil, stirring all the while. Salt to taste; let it boil a few minutes longer and take from the fire. Just before serving stir the prunes into the milk.

CHERRY SOUP.

Wash and pit sour cherries; boil them in a little water and sugar till done. Meanwhile, or the day before, soak stale bread in cold water till soft. Put this on a moderate fire, with the juice of one lemon and a little salt; boil ten minutes, stirring constantly; then put the cherries into it and set aside.

APPLE SOUP.

Two quarts of apples, ½ pint of white wine, water, sugar and instantaneous tapioca.

Cut the apples in pieces, unpeeled; wash them and boil them in a little water till well done. Put them through a sieve, pour water on this sauce and let them boil again for a few minutes. Stir 2 tablespoonfuls of tapioca, with the wine and sugar, into the soup and boil one or two minutes longer.

BUTTERMILK SOUP.

Cook 2 cups of pearl barley with ½ tablespoonful of flour till well done. Bring to a boil 1 quart of buttermilk with ½ tablespoonful of flour, stirring constantly. Add the barley and salt, sweeten to taste, and add 1 egg just before serving.

BARLEY SOUP.

One-half pound of prunes, 2 cups of barley. Boil each alone till well done in a little water; salt and sweeten to taste. Add a little butter and 1 quart of milk; bring to a boil together and take off.

RICE SOUP.

Put 4 ounces of rice in water and heat till just before the boiling point, then pour the water off and add fresh cold water to it. Boil slowly with 1 tablespoonful of butter till well done. Meanwhile stir 1 teaspoonful of flour in a cup of milk; pour this with some vegetable stock into the boiling rice, salt to taste and cook for 15 minutes longer, stirring all the while. Before serving add the yolks of 2 eggs.

QUAKER OATS SOUP.

One large cup of Quaker Oats, ¼ cup of butter, 1 quart of water, salt and vegetable stock.

After having melted the butter, stir the oats into it. When well mixed add the water, vegetable stock and salt; boil all till well done and serve. If desired any kind of fruit juice may be added to the soup.

FARINA SOUP.

Bring to a boil ½ pound of washed seedless raisins or ¼ pound of currants and raisins mixed, in a little water; season with a little lemon spice (see page 207) and salt. Add slowly while stirring constantly 1 cup of farina. Cook 10 minutes, take off, and just before serving add 1 egg, well beaten; sweeten to taste and flavor with juice of a lemon and a cup of cider.

This soup may be made with corn-meal, instantaneous tapioca, pearl barley, wheat hearts, gruenkorn or rice instead of farina.

BROWN SOUP.

In a deep dry pan, brown very evenly, stirring constantly, 1 cup of flour. When of a chocolate brown, pour cold water on it. Season with salt and 2 teaspoonfuls of butter and take off.

This soup is particularly good for convalescents.

CRANBERRY SOUP.

Take 6 cups of cranberry sauce; add to it 1 cup of gingerbread or ginger snaps soaked in water; add salt and sugar to taste and 1 teaspoonful of corn-starch dissolved in a little water, and boil awhile. Take off and serve with toast, crackers or breadsticks.

This soup may be made with muskmelon, raspberry sauce or goose-berry sauce instead of cranberries.

COLD SOUPS.

PEACH SOUP.

Peel and cut into pieces 2 pounds of very ripe peaches; sprinkle sugar over them and pour on a mixture of half cider and half water. Let them stand an hour and serve with vanilla wafers.

RASPBERRY SOUP.

Take 1 quart of raspberries; wash them if necessary and stir through a hair sieve; pour over them a mixture of 1 quart of water and the juice of 2 lemons. Sweeten to taste, put spiceless wafers in the tureen and pour the soup over them.

This soup may be made of blackberries instead of raspberries.

HUCKLEBERRY SOUP.

Wash 2 pounds of huckleberries; put them in water, bring to a boil and stir through a fine hair sieve into a bowl in which is 3 ounces of sugar and ½ bottle of cider. Serve with dice-shaped pieces of toast or breadsticks.

CLABBER SOUP.

Put fresh milk into a bowl in a moderately warm place for 1 or 2 days till it turns to clabber; sprinkle over it sugar and grated brown or graham bread, a little cinnamon and grated gingersnaps.

ALMOND MILK SOUP.

Take 4 ounces of sweet almonds and 8 ounces of bitter almonds; chop them fine, then boil them in 3 quarts of sweet milk, in which is 1 peach leaf or lemon spice to taste, for ½ hour; add a tablespoonful of corn-starch mixed in a little of the cold sweet milk, a little sugar and salt, and boil awhile. Stir into the soup the well-beaten yolks of 2 eggs. When cold take out the peach leaf, beat to a stiff froth the whites of 2 eggs and from a spoon drop lumps of the froth at regular distances over the top of the soup. Serve cold with crackers or toast. Very good.

VANILLA SOUP.

This is made like the above, except that vanilla is used for flavoring instead of a peach leaf and the almonds are omitted, while a little more corn-starch is used.

PECAN SOUP.

This may be made the same as the almond soup, except that pecans are used instead of almonds.

CURD SOUP.

Stir 1 pound of curd through a hair sieve and add 2½ ounces of sugar; pour into the curd 1 quart of cream, being careful to beat the curd hard and constantly while pouring in the cream, that it may be light and foamy. Serve with grated gingerbread or breadsticks.

RICE SOUP.

Blanch and chop fine 1½ ounces of pecans; boil them in 1 quart of milk for 10 minutes and add 1 cup of rice flour or rice meal. Let it boil slowly for awhile, take off and sweeten to taste. Before serving beat into it the yolks of 2 eggs.

INSTANTANEOUS TAPIOCA SOUP.

This soup is made the same way as the above, except that instead of rice, instantaneous tapioca may be used, omitting the pecans.

CIDER SOUP.

Take 1 bottle of cider and the same amount of water; add to this 1 cup of seedless raisins soaked in hot water, sugar to taste, the juice of 1 lemon, rind of ½ lemon, 2½ pounds of grated stale graham bread or whole wheat bread. Let it stand for two hours, stirring now and then.

BREAD.

SOFT OATMEAL BREAD.

Take 1 pint of oatmeal that is left from breakfast; stir into it ½ pint of scalded milk; when well mixed add ½ cup of yellow corn-meal. When partly cold add quickly the yolks of 3 eggs, and then stir in the well-beaten whites. Cover the bottom of the baking pan with chopped dates, pour over them the bread mixture and bake in a quick oven 30 minutes. It should be broken with a fork and taken out with a spoon.

MUSH GEMS.

Stir ¾ of a cup of corn-meal with a pint of hot milk and boil till smooth. Take from the fire, add the yolks of 4 eggs and then the well-beaten whites. Bake in greased gem pans in a moderate oven 20 minutes.

BREADSTICKS.

Sift into a large bowl a quart of whole wheat flour; rub into it two teaspoonfuls of good butter and salt until thoroughly mixed with the flour. Now stir briskly with a large spoon while pouring in with the other hand ½ pint of cold water. This must now be kneaded into a firm, smooth dough. Cut off a piece the size of a small fist and roll it on the breadboard until it is about the thickness of the little finger and cut it into five-inch lengths. Put all in a long baking pan, being careful that they do not touch each other, and bake 1 hour, turning occasionally with a fork. The colder the dough is while working the closer and more tender the breadsticks will be.

MUFFINS OF WHEAT FLOUR.

Mix together 2 tablespoonfuls of milk, 2 tablespoonfuls of butter, 2 teaspoonfuls of sugar, yolks of 2 eggs, 1 teaspoonful of salt, 2 teaspoonfuls of baking powder, and stir into it white flour enough to make a dough of proper consistency. Then beat the whites of the eggs, mix all together and put in a well-greased pan and bake in a hot oven.

CORN-MEAL MUFFINS.

These are made the same as white flour muffins, except that more corn-meal and less white flour is used—about ⅔ corn-meal and ⅓ white flour.

CORN BREAD.

Make this the same as corn-meal muffins, but instead of baking in muffin pans bake in a long pan and when done cut into squares.

RYE BREAD.

Dissolve in the evening 1 compressed yeast cake in a quart of warm water; mix this with 4 teaspoonfuls of salt and as much rye flour as will make a stiff mass; stir it well and place during the night in a warm place to rise. In the morning knead it well for 1½ hours with wheat flour, form the dough into loaves, put in a warm place to rise again and bake them for 1½ hours in a good hot oven. It ought to have a good brown crust.

WHOLE WHEAT BREAD.

This is made like the above, except a little less wheat flour is used.

VEGETABLES.

VEGETABLE RAGOUT.

This is made of equal parts of boiled Irish potatoes cut in small square pieces, raw apples, cooked beets (cut fine), and a few seedless raisins.

Make a gravy of 1 tablespoonful of white flour, 1 tablespoonful of butter, and let it come to a boil; add salt and water, and put the vegetables, with Dr. Lahmann's naehrsalz (see page 206), and juice of ½ lemon into it and let all some to a boil again before serving.

CABBAGE WITH APPLES.

Chop ½ of a large cabbage very fine; boil it in a very little water with a little salt, good drippings and ½ tablespoonful of butter. When half done, add three large or five small cooking apples (peeled and sliced) to the cabbage, and cook till they are done. Pour over it the juice of ½ lemon and a little flour mixed together, and let boil awhile longer.

Red cabbage may also be used for a change in the same way.

CABBAGE WITH POTATOES.

Clean the cabbage leaves and cut in large pieces like lettuce and put with the necessary amount of boiling water on the fire till done; then peel and cut in pieces some Irish potatoes and add them to the cabbage and let them boil till done; season with good drippings, butter and salt; strew over a little flour, mix all well together, adding water when necessary; put in some beef drippings and let it boil for a few minutes longer.

SAUERKRAUT.

Put ⅔ ounce of butter or konut in a pot with a little boiling water; add 1 pound of sauerkraut and boil till done; then add ⅔ ounce of beef drippings, a few small cooked Irish potatoes, a little flour and Lahmann's nachrsalz (as much as 3 peas); put this with the cabbage, with the necessary amount of water, and mix well together.

SPINACH.

Take a peck of spinach and wash clean; put it in a very little boiling water, adding water when necessary. When well done take up, and if so preferred chop fine; this is a matter of taste. Make a gravy of 10 ounces of butter, with chopped onion and bread crumbs. Put the spinach into it and add sweet milk to taste.

Beet leaves may be used in the same way.

ONIONS.

Peel the onions and put them on the fire with butter, salt, a little nutmeg and grated zwieback; add a little water when necessary; flavor with lemon juice to taste and serve when done.

CARROTS.

After having cleaned and washed 2 bunches of carrots, cut them in small thin strips about 2 inches long and put them, with a tablespoonful of butter or konut, with a little water on a moderate fire, and when done sprinkle over the carrots a little flour, salt and sugar to taste, and chopped parsley. Let all boil together in the necessary amount of water slowly for a few minutes.

GREEN BEANS.

Two quarts of green beans. Break the beans in two or three pieces. After having washed the beans put them with ½ tablespoonful of beef drippings with a cupful of boiling water and boil till done. Meanwhile make a gravy of ½ tablespoonful of butter, 1 tablespoonful of flour, ½ chopped onion and the necessary amount of water, and salt to taste. Put the beans into it and let all come to a boil again.

15

WHITE BEANS.

After having shelled 2 quarts of beans, boil in a little water for several hours till done; then make a gravy with a little butter, ¼ tablespoonful of flour, salt and water and add to the beans. Pour over the beans a little milk, so they will not be too dry.

CUT BEANS.

String very young green beans and cut them in thin lengthwise pieces; wash these and mix with them butter, salt, ½ onion, chopped fine, and a very little water. Boil until done, adding water to them when necessary. Mix a little flour in with the beans and boil together.

BEETS.

Boil the beets till done, but do not stick them with a fork or they will lose their fine red color. Then cut in round slices and add butter and a little lemon juice.

KOHLRABI.

Peel and cut 1 peck of kohlrabi in round fine slices and boil in a little water till done. Take off and cool, and if there is too much water pour off in another pan. Then make a gravy with this water, 1 pint of milk, salt, Lahmann's naehrsalz, ½ tablespoonful of flour and a tablespoonful of butter; add this gravy to the kohlrabi and let all come to a boil again. If the kohlrabi is young and has greens, cut and boil both together.

WHITE TURNIPS.

Take ½ peck of nice, sweet, white turnips; peel and cut them in pieces; make a gravy of 1 tablespoonful of good beef drippings or butter, milk and salt and put the turnips into it; bring all to a boil till well done, and add as often as necessary a little milk or cream, and mix well together before serving.

WAX BEANS.

These beans are to be cooked just like the green beans, except that milk instead of water is used and the onions are omitted.

CAULIFLOWER.

Cut off the stalks and take out the little leaves with a small knife, so that the head of the cauliflower does not break in pieces; put it in cold water awhile to clean, and then put it on the fire with a little salt in the water and boil till done; pour off the water, which is to be saved for the sauce, and serve with cream, sauce or melted butter.

TURNIP GREENS WITH POTATOES.

Strip the leaves of a bucketful of turnip greens from the stems; wash these well and cut them fine; put with ½ pint of water on the fire together with a piece of bacon and some salt; boil till nearly done; then add a large grated raw potato and ½ cup of milk and let boil 15 or 20 minutes longer. Must not be watery but fluid evaporated.

GERMAN KALE.

Wash and cut the kale and boil in ½ pint of water till half done. Meanwhile cook in another pot a piece of beef, ham or bacon; when done mix it with the kale and sprinkle a little flour over it. Mix well, let the fluid evaporate and serve.

CAULIFLOWER WITH CHEESE.

After having cooked the cauliflower as in the above "plain cauliflower," serve nicely in a deep dish; mix the cream sauce with 1 or 2 tablespoonfuls of grated Parmesan or Swiss cheese; pour it over the cauliflower and cover entirely with cheese and melted butter and brown in a hot oven.

OYSTER PLANT.

Take a tablespoonful of flour and mix well with water or milk; clean each piece of the oyster plant in hot water and peel; cut in 2 or 3 lengths and boil in the above gravy till done; add the necessary amount of butter, salt and sugar, and before serving sprinkle with bread crumbs.

ASPARAGUS.

Peel the asparagus from head to end and cut off as much as is hard; wash and tie in small bundles; put in boiling water enough to cover and boil very slowly, otherwise the softer parts will cook to pieces before the rest. Season with a very little salt, so as not to harden the asparagus. Serve with melted butter or asparagus gravy.

MUSHROOMS.

Cut off a little piece from the ends, wash them carefully and put them on the fire with butter and a little water; let them boil slowly ½ hour, then add a teaspoonful of white flour or grated zwieback, a little salt and lemon juice to the gravy and thicken with the yolk of an egg.

CHESTNUTS.

Peel the chestnuts, pour hot water over them and take off the inner skin; season with a little salt, sugar and butter and boil till done; then add a little flour and mix together.

DRIED WHITE BEANS.

Soak them over night in cold water, then put on the fire and boil; change the water twice, then add good beef drippings, a little salt, and when well done, before serving, add lemon juice to taste.

DRIED PEAS.

Soak and cook the peas the same as white dried beans. When done stir through a sieve, season with salt and good beef drippings. Before serving pour over them a gravy of chopped onions browned in butter. The peas are to be thickened and are good eaten with sauerkraut.

DRIED GREEN BEANS IN THE SHELL.

Dry small green beans in the shell during the autumn for winter use. Before using soak over night in cold water, and then boil in fresh water till done. Add water when necessary, season with salt and lemon juice to taste, and let all boil together for awhile.

LENTILS.

Put the lentils in cold water to boil till done. Then brown a little cut onion and flour in drippings and butter and mix with hot water. Stir this into the lentils and add salt to taste.

POTATO DISHES.

POTATOES WITH MILK SAUCE.

Take medium-sized potatoes; peel and boil till done; add the salt just before done, in order not to harden them, so they will not fall to pieces; pour off the water, make a milk sauce and pour over before serving. Make plentifully of the sauce, as good mealy potatoes are very absorbent.

SOUR POTATOES.

Make good beef drippings very hot; brown in it some fine chopped onions and thicken with a little flour; add the potatoes with water and salt and boil till done. Serve with lemon juice to taste.

MASHED POTATOES.

Boil the potatoes in salted water and put through a sieve; add butter and milk, or milk and boiling water, till the potatoes are of the right consistency. If agreeable, onions chopped fine or zwieback browned in hot butter may be stirred into the mashed potatoes.

POTATO SLICES FRIED.

Peel the potatoes, wash and cut in thin round or lengthwise slices, then put half butter and half beef drippings in a pan and put the potatoes in it; sprinkle with salt, pour over a cup of water and cover; then let them cook till done and fry a yellow brown.

POTATOES WITH APPLES.

Cook some Irish potatoes alone; also alone the same amount of sour apples; then mix both together well, mashing as in mashed potatoes; add salt, good beef drippings, butter and a little sugar to taste, and let them come to a boil. Before serving pour over them a thick sauce made of grated zwieback in melted butter.

SALADS.

In making a salad it is always best to pour the olive oil over the salad and then mix in the other ingredients.

LETTUCE.

Clean, cut and wash the lettuce well in cold water. Just before serving mix with juice of ½ lemon, a little salt and ½ onion, chopped fine.

WATER CRESS.

Prepare just like lettuce; and add hard-boiled eggs chopped fine.

BEAN SALAD.

Clean fine green beans; boil till done, then pour off the water and when cool mix with salt, lemon juice, olive oil and an onion chopped fine.

MIXED SALADS.

Take equal portions of cold sliced Irish potatoes and beets, and add sliced apples or red cabbage, chopped fine, and salted cucumbers; mix all together (being very careful not to break the slices) with oil, salt, lemon juice and juice of the beets.

POTATO SALAD.

Cook Irish potatoes with the peel, using a kind that are not too mealy; cut them in thin slices, mix with a little hot water, salt, lemon juice, an onion chopped fine, or sour cream.

Salads may be made in the same way of beans and cucumbers.

SALAD OF WHITE OR RED CABBAGE.

Chop the cabbage very fine; mix with sour cream sauce and serve with potatoes.

VEGETABLE SALAD.

Take 1 part of cauliflower, 1 part of carrots, 1 part of peas and 1 part of asparagus tips, and boil each ingredient separately till done; then mix lightly, put on a large flat plate, cover with mayonnaise sauce and serve.

CUCUMBER SALAD.

Wash, peel and slice the cucumbers very thin; just before serving pour over them olive oil, salt and lemon juice, or if preferred take 1 hard-boiled egg, mash it up very fine with a fork and then stir into it olive oil, salt, lemon juice or sour cream, and mix in with the cucumbers.

CELERY SALAD.

Wash and clean the celery and cut it into 1 or 2-inch lengths; then mix it with mayonnaise sauce.

DUMPLINGS.

The white bread which is for dumplings need not be fresh nor put in warm or hot water; use stale, soak it in cold water and press out the surplus water.

FINE POTATO DUMPLINGS.

Take 2 soup plates full of grated potatoes which have been cooked the day before in the peel; add 3 tablespoonfuls of flour, a little nutmeg, salt, a small cup of butter, Lahmann's naehrsalz and 4 or 5 eggs; the whites and yolks must be well beaten separately, the whites to a stiff froth; mix all together well; dip out with a table-spoon and drop into boiling salted water and boil 15 minutes. Serve with melted butter.

RICE DUMPLINGS.

Wash ½ pound of best rice; put it in cold water and boil slowly till well done; let it cool; add 4 eggs, salt, Lahmann's naehrsalz, 2 ounces of butter well beaten with 1 tablespoonful of flour; form into small dumplings and cook them in boiling water. Serve with tomato sauce.

CLABBER DUMPLINGS.

Mix 1 pint of clabber with 1 pint of grated potatoes, cooked the day before; add 2 eggs, 4 ounces of flour, salt and caraway seeds to taste. When well mixed, boil all together in salted boiling water.

PANCAKES.

Pancakes are to be fried in equal parts of Ko-nut and butter, which makes them more easily digested, and they are not so apt to burn in frying.

POTATO PANCAKES.

Peel, wash and grate raw Irish potatoes; add salt, 2 or 3 eggs, an onion chopped fine, Lahmann's nachrsalz. Mix all well together and bake in little, round, thin cakes in hot Ko-nut and butter.

EGG PANCAKES.

For 3 large cakes which fill the pan, take the yolks of 6 fresh eggs, 6 small spoonfuls of flour, 1 pint of sweet milk, 2 pints of sour cream and a little salt.

Beat the yolks of the eggs, cream, flour and salt together well, then stir in the milk. Just before baking add the well-beaten whites of the eggs.

CORN-STARCH PANCAKES.

Take yolks of 4 eggs, 2 ounces of corn-starch, 1 pint of warm milk, ½ pint of water and a little salt; beat all well together; add the well-beaten whites and bake in hot butter and Ko-nut.

FLOUR PANCAKES.

For a medium-sized pancake, which covers the pan, take ⅛ pound of flour, 2 eggs, 1 pint of milk and a little salt. Beat all well together and bake in hot butter and Ko-nut.

CURRANT PANCAKES.

Three eggs, 2½ tablespoonfuls of flour, 1 pint of sweet milk, mixed with a little water, a little salt and sugar. Beat well. Put Ko-nut and butter in a pan. When hot, put in the batter; pour over it the washed currants with sugar to taste. Before turning pour over the currants fine grated zwieback, and serve on this side sprinkled with sugar.

SOUR CHERRY PANCAKES.

May be made the same as above, except that cherries are used instead of currants.

APPLE PANCAKES.

Peel and cut in thin slices a soup-plateful of nice ripe apples. Put in a pan and cover with a little butter; pour over them the batter (as in currant pancake); let them bake till done. Turn and bake without zwieback. Serve with sugar sprinkled over them.

PANCAKES WITH SWEET CORN.

Make a batter as above and mix in it fresh sweet corn left from dinner. Bake in little cakes on both sides in Ko-nut. Serve with maple syrup.

BUCKWHEAT PANCAKES.

To every cup of buckwheat flour take 1 cup of hot water, 1 cup of sour cream or a little Ko-nut or butter, a little salt and ¼ ounce yeast; dried currants may also be added. After having beaten all thoroughly together, set the batter aside to rise. When light, bake like other pancakes.

VEGETABLE SLICES.

GRUENKORN SLICES.

Take 1½ cups of gruenkorn; put with it 1 tablespoonful of butter, a little salt and a little cold water, and boil five or six hours, till soft. Use as little water as possible, being careful, however, that it does not burn. When done take off and cool. Meanwhile chop an onion fine and fry it in melted butter; add this with 2 eggs, a little bread crumbs, salt and Lahmann's naehrsalz to the gruenkorn. Cut in slices, turn in bread crumbs and fry on both sides in hot Ko-nut. Serve with onion gravy. Very good and nourishing.

MUSH SLICES.

Use mush, grits, oatmeal or flakes for this nice supper dish; 1½ cups of cereal; boil till done. Mix with 1 or 2 eggs, salt, Lahmann's naehrsalz and a little nutmeg. Cut in slices and bake like pancakes with sweet corn.

SLICES OF VEGETABLES.

Take cold, cooked vegetables, such as spinach, carrots, peas or beans; chop them, add salt, 3 or 4 eggs, chopped onion and grated bread crumbs. Fix them the same as other slices and fry in Ko-nut.

PEA SLICES.

Two cups of dried green peas, soaked over night in cold water. Boil till done, stir through a sieve, add little pieces of white bread, chopped onion heated in melted butter, and 2 or 3 eggs. Cover with grated bread crumbs and fry in Ko-nut and butter.

TOMATO SLICES.

One dinner-plateful of cooked and grated potatoes, the same amount of peeled sliced tomatoes, 3 ounces of butter, 2 eggs, salt and Lahmann's naehrsalz. Mix well together and then bake like the other slices.

VARIOUS DINNER AND SUPPER DISHES.

SOUR CREAM DISH.

Beat ¼ pound of butter with 1 quart of sour cream till foamy, then add the yolks of 6 eggs, a little salt, ½ pound of grated white bread, and lastly the stiff beaten whites of the eggs. Bake in a china baking dish in a hot oven for 1 hour.

CORN-MEAL.

Pour ¼ pound of white corn-meal in 1 quart of boiling water, and let it cook slowly for awhile; take off, and when cool add the yolks of 4 eggs, a little salt, Lahmann's naehrsalz and, lastly, the well-beaten whites. Put it in a well-greased pan, cover with butter and grated bread crumbs and boil in hot water.

GRUENKORN.

Boil ¼ pound of grated gruenkorn with 1 pint of milk slowly till done. Meanwhile soak 3 large zwiebacks, or the same amount of stale white bread without the crust, in water. Fry 1 onion, chopped fine, in 1 large tablespoonful of butter till brown. Press out the zwieback or bread from the water and mix it well with the corn. Stir in the yolks of 3 eggs, add Lahmann's naehrsalz, salt to taste and add a little nutmeg, and finally the well-beaten whites of the eggs. Mix all together thoroughly and put in a pan well greased and lined with bread crumbs, and boil 1¼ hours.

MUSHROOMS.

Peel, cut and soak 4 zwiebacks, or the same amount of white bread, in water. Press the water from the zwieback or bread and put it in a pan with a tablespoonful of butter, chopped onion, parsley, salt and Lahmann's naehrsalz. Set it on the stove and let it brown for awhile. Meanwhile chop fine ½ pound of good mushrooms, stew them till tender in a little butter, take off and add 4 yolks of eggs, finally the well-beaten whites of the eggs, and cook all together in a good gravy. Put all in a pan, well greased and lined with bread crumbs, and boil for 1 hour in hot water.

TAPIOCA.

Put ¼ pound of instantaneous tapioca with 1 large tablespoonful of butter in 1 pint of boiling water till thick and well done. When cool add the well-beaten yolks of 4 or 5 eggs, 1 teacupful of flour and a little nutmeg to taste. Finally add the well-beaten whites of the eggs and cook like the above.

SPINACH.

Take 1 can of spinach, or the fresh (preferred); chop it a little, with 1 onion, a little parsley and a little salt. Stew it with 1 table-spoonful of butter. Meanwhile soak 4 or 5 zwiebacks in milk. Press out the milk, mix it with 2½ ounces of butter, which has been beaten to a cream, and with all the above ingredients. Finally, stir in the well-beaten whites of the eggs and put all in a well-greased pan lined with bread crumbs. Cook 1 hour in boiling water, or bake in a china bake dish in the oven.

QUAKER OATS.

Beat 6 ounces of butter to a cream; add to it the yolks of 4 or 5 eggs and 3 ounces of Quaker Oats. Then cook 3 large tablespoonfuls of vegetables, such as cauliflower or asparagus, in a little water till done. Pour off the water and mix it with the whites of the eggs; season with a little salt. Mix all together and bake like the above.

RICE DISH.

Boil ½ pound best rice in a little water till about half done; then pour off the water. Put a little butter in a pan, add to it 1½ quarts of milk and ½ quart of water and let it come to a boil. Put the rice in it and cook till done, neither too stiff nor too soft. Add to taste a little salt and sugar. Serve cold or warm.

RICE WITH APPLES.

Boil ½ pound of best rice with 1 quart of milk till about half done. Put a little butter in a pan, put the rice in, add boiling water and let it cook slowly. When nearly done, add peeled and sliced apples, and sugar to taste; let all boil together. When necessary shake, but do not stir, so as not to break the rice. Sprinkle sugar over it and serve.

TOAST AND CHEESE.

Grate Edam or Swiss cheese and mix with the same amount of butter to a cream, and spread on nicely toasted white bread. Serve hot or cold.

PARSLEY ON TOAST.

Cream 3 ounces of butter, add juice of 1 lemon and 3 tablespoonfuls of parsley, chopped fine. Mix well together and spread on cold buttered toast.

MUSHROOMS ON TOAST.

Stew two tablespoonfuls of best mushrooms with a little water and butter. Then put it through a sieve. Beat 3 ounces of butter to a cream, mix it with the mushrooms, stew again and spread on toast or white bread.

CLABBER CREAM.

Beat clabber with the cream for 15 minutes. Sweeten to taste, flavor with cinnamon and fruit juice and serve with crackers.

EGGS.

SCRAMBLED EGGS.

Take to each person 1 egg, 1 tablespoonful of milk, a little salt and ½ tablespoonful of butter. Beat eggs, milk, butter and salt together and cook in melted butter. As soon as it thickens, dip out with a spoon in small slices, put in a dish and serve. Instead of butter, some prefer to use water in mixing.

DROPPED EGGS.

Bring to a boil 1 quart of water and 1 pint of lemon juice and a little salt. The eggs are to be cooked in this one at a time. Drop an egg in, take a large spoon, and, with this, carefully keep the white covered over the yolk. When the white hardens take the egg out and pour cold water over it.

OMELETTE.

Take 1 tablespoonful of flour and dissolve it in 2 tablespoonfuls of tepid milk and the yolks of 4 eggs, a little salt and sugar, and stir all thoroughly together. Finally add the whites beaten to a snow. Bake in a batter pan slowly on one side till the dough looks dry; put on a platter and sprinkle over the half of it the juice of a lemon and some sugar. Double over and sprinkle over with sugar.

OMELETTE WITH JELLY.

Bake an omelette like the above, omitting the lemon juice. When taken up spread raspberry or apple jelly over it. Double over and serve hot.

EGGS IN CUPS.

Grease the earthenware egg cups with melted butter. Break into each cup 2 eggs; sprinkle with a little salt; have a pan of boiling water on the stove; set the egg cups in, letting the water cover the cups as high as the eggs in the cups. Let them stay 8 minutes in the water. Take out, let them cool in the cups and turn out, or serve hot in the cups.

MEATS.

BEEF ROAST.

Put beef drippings in a pan on the top of the stove; beat the beef, rub salt in on both sides; add it then to the drippings with sliced onions, and a little garlic to taste. Let fry on both sides, keeping closely covered all the time. Then put in an oven to bake and pour the gravy over it every 10 minutes, keeping covered well between times. A roast of 5 pounds will need to be covered nearly 3 hours. When done take out and sprinkle flour in the gravy to thicken it, and if necessary add a little hot water and boil a few minutes.

VEAL ROAST.

For this roast take, instead of beef drippings, butter and a little bacon, without onions or garlic. Cook in the same way as the beef roast, but only two hours. Add finally the gravy with a little sour cream or milk.

MUTTON ROAST.

Rub salt into the roast and cook the same as the beef roast.

RABBIT STEW.

Wash and cut the meat into small pieces; put in a china dish and pour over it boiled cider or lemon juice and water in which is cut onions, spices and bay leaves. Let the meat stay in this spiced vinegar 1 or 2 days. Then take out, put in a pan on the stove with a little of the cider, adding water, fresh-cut onions, a little salt and flour and boil till done. Finally thicken the gravy with browned flour, add white wine and a very little sugar to taste.

COLD MEAT JELLY.

Take of pig's feet and calf's feet an equal number; cook them till done in a little water, with salt, cut onions, spices and lemon juice to taste. Take up when done and empty all into a sieve, saving the gravy which is drained from the meat. Cut the meat from the feet in small dice-shaped pieces and put in the gravy to cook again till well done. Then pour very cold water in a china dish and empty it out again, not drying, as this prevents sticking. Pour the meat and gravy into the wet dish, being sure to have gravy enough to cover the meat. Let it stand till it is stiff, then cut in slices and serve plain, or it is very nice with mayonnaise sauce.

FRIED CHICKEN.

Clean and wash the chicken without cutting it up; rub some salt over it and fry in butter in an open pan till it is a light brown on both sides. Then add a little water, put in the oven and baste every 10 minutes with the gravy. Keep covered, and when done take out of the gravy and carve just before serving. Thicken the gravy with a little flour and boil a few minutes.

STEWED CHICKEN.

Wash and clean the chicken, cut it in pieces and cook till nearly done in boiling salted water. Put some butter and flour (1 tablespoonful for each chicken) in a pot; add to this a part of the gravy in which the chicken was cooked, and the chicken, and boil together till done. Then take out the chicken and stir into the gravy the beaten yolk of an egg; pour the gravy over the chicken and serve with cooked rice around the dish.

STEWED VEAL.

This is cooked like the stewed chicken, except that, before well done, a fine chopped onion and capers to taste is added.

SAUCES FOR MEATS AND VEGETABLES.

SOUR EGG SAUCE FOR GREEN BEANS AND POTATOES.

Beat the yolks of 2 eggs with 2 tablespoonfuls of best flour and 1 pint of fresh milk; add ½ tablespoonful of good butter, a little grated nutmeg and lemon juice to give a sour taste. Put on the fire with a little salt, stir continually till done and sufficiently thickened.

CAULIFLOWER SAUCE.

Take fresh butter, melt it and add to it ½ tablespoonful of flour, a little fresh milk, salt and nutmeg; beat all well together on the fire till thick; take off and add the well-beaten yolks of 2 eggs.

ASPARAGUS SAUCE.

Take yolks of 3 eggs, 1½ tablespoonfuls of flour, 3 tablespoonfuls of sweet cream, 1 pint of asparagus water, or plain water, a little nutmeg, juice of 1½ lemons and sugar to taste. Beat all together and stir on the fire till it thickens. Take off and stir in ½ tablespoonful of butter and salt to taste.

FINE ONION SAUCE.

Peel and cut 3 or 4 onions in small pieces and fry them in a pan with a little piece of fat and 1 tablespoonful of flour till brown; then add as much water as is required for the desired amount, and boil slowly for awhile. Stir through a sieve and bring again to a boil, with a little nutmeg and salt. Take off and stir into it a fresh piece of butter, the yolk of an egg and a little of Liebig's extract of beef.

This sauce is suitable for boiled meats or potatoes.

MAYONNAISE SAUCE.

Beat 2 or 3 yolks of fresh eggs, always in one direction; then add ½ small cup of olive oil, pouring it in by drops and beating all the while in the same direction, till the sauce is thick. Add salt to taste.

CREAM SAUCE FOR SALADS.

Beat well some thick sour cream with lemon juice, fine olive oil, a little salt, and, to taste, a little fine chopped onion.

PARSLEY SAUCE.

Chop the parsley fine and stew it in 3 ounces of butter, 2 tablespoonfuls of flour, for 5 or 6 minutes; then add as much water as desired.

MUSHROOM SAUCE.

Take 4 ounces of butter, 3 tablespoonfuls of flour and dissolve in water; let it stew for awhile, then add the juice of 1 lemon, ½ chopped onion, a little nutmeg and salt. Meanwhile boil the mushrooms in salted water till done; chop them fine and mix with the other ingredients, adding lemon juice to taste.

CUCUMBER SAUCE.

Chop 1 onion fine; stew it in 4 ounces of butter; add cucumbers, peeled and cut in very small squares; let them stew together for a few minutes, then sprinkle 2½ tablespoonfuls of flour over them and add water, a little sour cream, salt, Lahmann's naehrsalz and the juice of 1 lemon, and let all boil well together.

16

SWEET SAUCES.

STRAWBERRY SAUCE.

Stir 1 pint of strawberry marmalade through a sieve; add 1 quart of water and lemon juice to taste. If the sauce is desired thicker, stir into the boiling juice 1 tablespoonful of corn-starch dissolved in water and boil again a few moments.

RASPBERRY SAUCE.

Boil fresh raspberries with water; stir through a sieve; mix with water and flavor with lemon juice to taste.

CHERRY SAUCE.

Let 1 quart of sour cherries come to a boil with 1 quart of water and stir through a hair sieve; put the juice again on the stove; add sugar to taste and 1 tablespoonful of corn-starch dissolved in water; let all come to a boil together and serve hot or cold.

PRUNE SAUCE. No. 1.

Wash fresh prunes, stone them and boil with water; when done stir through a hair sieve; put the juice again on the fire, add the necessary sugar and corn-starch and let it come to a boil.

PRUNE SAUCE. No. 2.

Stone ½ pound dried prunes; wash and boil till done in 1 quart of water, then stir through a sieve. Add to this the pulp, juice and peel of 1 lemon and sugar to taste, and put on the fire to boil. If not thick enough, stir in a little dissolved corn-starch.

APPLE SAUCE.

Peel and cut the apples in pieces; 1 quart of water, 1 soup-plateful of sliced apples, add a few slices of lemon, ½ tablespoonful of butter, and boil till done; stir through a sieve and add ½ cup of washed and boiled currants and a little dissolved corn-starch.

Prune and apple sauce are nice to serve with dumplings.

CRANBERRY SAUCE.

Boil nice ripe cranberries in water till done, and stir through a sieve; add to this sugar and lemon juice to taste.

FRUIT FOAM.

Beat the whites of 4 or 5 eggs stiff and mix with 1 quart of fruit juice; add sugar and lemon juice to taste.

RED CURRANT SAUCE.

Stir 1 pint of washed and cooked currants through a sieve. Add to the juice ½ pound of sugar; beat together for 15 minutes and serve with cold rice and blanc-mange.

FOAM SAUCE.

Take ½ bottle of unfermented grape juice, yolks of 3 fresh eggs and 2 whole eggs, ½ tablespoonful of best flour, 2½ ounces of sugar, juice and peel of 1 lemon; put all together in a steam pot on the fire and stir until the fluid is foamy.

VANILLA SAUCE.

Bring 1 quart of milk, with sugar and vanilla, to a boil, then beat well the yolks of 6 eggs with a little milk (saved from the quart); stir this into the boiling milk, beating well on the fire for awhile, but take off before it comes again to a boil.

CHOCOLATE SAUCE.

Put 3 ounces of chocolate in a very little water on the fire to dissolve; add 1 pint of cream and 1 pint of sweet milk, a little vanilla and sugar to taste. Take off and beat in the yolks of 2 eggs.

COMPOTES.

Be careful in cooking fruits to stir without breaking them. Boil them always on a moderate fire with a little sugar and a little water.

GOOSEBERRY COMPOTE.

Clean the green gooseberries from the stems, etc.; wash them and boil them in a little water, adding water when necessary; add sugar and white wine to taste and boil till done. Then stir in 2 eggs well beaten and take off.

HUCKLEBERRY COMPOTE.

Take 2 quarts of huckleberries, clean and wash them, and boil with water and sugar. Pour a layer of them in a china dish and on this a layer of zwieback and continue this till the dish is full. Serve cold.

APPLE COMPOTE.

Peel and cut good ripe sour apples and boil with water, sugar and dried currants. The currants and apple slices must remain whole. When soft, take carefully out of the juice, which is to be boiled again with the juice of a lemon, and pour over the compote. Let it cool and serve.

RHUBARB COMPOTE.

Peel the rhubarb stalks and cut in 2-inch pieces. Boil slowly till soft in a little water, with sugar and lemon juice to taste. Use 1 glass of water and 4 ounces of sugar to every ½ pound of cut rhubarb.

STRAWBERRY COMPOTE.

Clean and wash 1 quart of ripe strawberries; cover with 6 ounces of sugar and let stand several hours; drain off the juice through a colander, add more sugar to the juice, according to taste, and let it boil till stiff. Let it cool and then pour over the strawberries.

PLUM COMPOTE.

Wash and stone nice ripe plums or prunes; put in a dish with a very little water and a good deal of sugar; cover closely and put in the oven to stew for ½ hour. Then serve with the juice (cold) in a glass dish.

RED CURRANT COMPOTE.

Bring some sugar and water to a boil; add to it the washed and cleaned currants; take off and pour into a colander; take the juice which is drained off, add more sugar to it and let it boil till it thickens. When cool, pour over the currants.

MIXED FRUIT COMPOTE.

Take equal quantities of currants, strawberries and cherries; bring each kind to a boil separately in sugar and water. When done, mix together and serve with crackers.

PEACH COMPOTE.

Make a syrup of sugar and water; add the peeled fruit and let it boil slowly till done, being careful to keep the fruit whole. Take off and serve when cool.

PRUNE MARMALADE.

Five ounces dried prunes, 2 ounces dried peaches and 2 ounces dried apples. Bring each kind to a boil separately till done. Stir through a sieve and put all together with sugar and lemon juice on the fire to boil for awhile.

PEAR COMPOTE.

Peel the pears, cut in halves and take out the cores, and then put them in water. Meanwhile put a little butter and sugar in a pan on the stove. Add the pears out of the water and let stew for awhile till they begin to brown, then sprinkle over them some sugar; cover up again until they are a nice brown.

WARM PUDDINGS.

The success of a pudding depends largely upon the thorough creaming of the butter and the beating of the eggs, whites and yolks separately, and the whites always to be added last, beaten as stiff as possible.

The forms or molds in which the warm puddings are to be baked or boiled must first be well greased with butter and then thickly sprinkled over with very finely grated bread crumbs. This prevents the pudding from sticking to the mold and forms an agreeable crust.

Before using corn-starch always dissolve it in a little cold water or milk.

RICE PUDDING.

One-quarter pound best rice, 1 pint of milk, grated peel of lemon and juice of ½ lemon, 2 ounces of butter, 2 ounces of sugar and 4 or 5 eggs.

Soak the rice, pour off the water and boil in milk, flavored with lemon peel, till done; let it cool, then add the butter beaten to a cream, the sugar, the yolk of the eggs and the lemon juice, and lastly the whites of the eggs beaten stiff. Put this mixture and macaroons in layers in a pudding mold and boil in hot water 2½ hours. This is for 4 to 6 persons.

SAGO PUDDING.

One-half pound of best sago, cooked in milk till thick; 5 eggs, 2½ ounces of butter, 2½ ounces of sugar, 2 ounces grated zwieback, 1 cup of sweet cream and the grated peel of 1 lemon. Mix and cook like rice pudding.

VANILLA PUDDING.

Three-quarters of a pound of stale bread without the crust, 1 pint of fresh cream or milk, 2 ounces butter, 2½ ounces grated almonds, 2½ ounces sugar, 5 or 6 eggs and vanilla to taste.

Soak the bread in the milk, cream the butter and add the yolks of the eggs, almonds, sugar and vanilla. Beat all the ingredients together for 15 minutes, always in the same direction, and lastly, add the stiff-beaten whites of the eggs. Boil 1½ or 2 hours, and serve with fruit juice sauce.

ZWIEBACK PUDDING.

Three ounces of zwieback, 1 cup seedless raisins, 5 eggs, ¾ quart of fresh milk, 1½ or 2 ounces sugar and a little nutmeg or vanilla to taste.

Put some zwieback, several hours before cooking, in the bottom of a pudding mold. Beat the eggs, whites and yolks together, add them to the other ingredients and pour a layer of the batter over the zwieback and then put in a layer of the zwieback, etc., till all ingredients are in, in this way, finishing with the zwieback. Boil 1½ or 2 hours, and bake in a china dish 1 hour.

BREAD PUDDING WITH ALMONDS.

One-half pound stale sifted rye bread crumbs or whole wheat bread, ¼ pound of butter, 8 eggs, ½ pound sugar, ¼ pound grated almonds, grated peel of 1 lemon and the juice of 3 or 4 lemons.

Stir the bread in with the butter on the fire, add the lemon juice, take off and let it cool. Then add all the ingredients and finally the stiff-beaten whites of the eggs. Boil the pudding 2 or 2½ hours, or bake 1¼ hours. Serve with hot or cold fruit sauce. For 12 or 14 persons.

CHOCOLATE PUDDING.

One quart of milk, ¼ pound white flour, 4 ounces butter, ¼ pound unsweetened chocolate, ¼ pound sugar, ¼ pound almonds and 5 eggs.

Boil the chocolate with the butter and flour; take off, add the almonds, sugar, yolks of the eggs and finally the stiff-beaten whites. Put all in a form which has been greased with butter, and sprinkle with grated zwieback and bake for 1 hour. Serve with vanilla sauce.

FRUIT PUDDING.

Two pounds stale white bread or zwieback, 1 quart of milk, ¼ pound butter, 8 or 10 eggs, 6 or 8 ounces sugar, fruit (such as sour apples or cherries), lemon peel, lemon juice to taste and ¼ pound dried currants.

Cut tbe bread in small pieces without tbe crust, mix witb tbe butter and milk and stir in a pan on the stove till it comes from the sides of the pan. Let cool; add all the other ingredients and lastly the stiff-beaten wbites of the eggs. Put a layer of the batter in a pan, spread a layer of fruit over this and then a layer of the batter, etc., until all the ingredients are used, ending with the batter on top. Cook for 2 hours. For 12 or 14 persons.

MACAROON PUDDING.

Cut the macaroons in pieces and put in a pudding mold which has been well greased; then strew in washed, soaked seedless raisins; pour over all 4 or 5 well-beaten eggs with 3 pints of milk, 2 ounces of sugar and bake or boil 1 hour.

ORANGE PUDDING.

One-quarter pound white corn-meal, 2 ounces butter, 4 ounces sugar, 3 pints of milk, 5 eggs and 3 oranges.

Let the butter and milk come to a boil; stir into it the meal and cook till done. Take off and let it cool, then add sugar, the yolks of the eggs, the juice and grated peel of 1 orange. Peel the other 2 oranges and lay the sections on the bottom of a well-greased pan. Cover all witb the batter and bake for ¾ of an bour.

GOOSEBERRY PUDDING.

One-balf pound green gooseberries, ½ pound sugar, ½ pound grated white bread or zwieback, 6 ounces butter, 6 or 8 eggs, 3 pints of milk.

Boil the gooseberries witb half the sugar and a little water till done; take off and let it stand a day, then toast tbe bread in tbe butter to a light brown; add the milk and boil together till stiff; after it is cool add the well-beaten yolks of the eggs, the rest of tbe sugar and the gooseberries without the juice, and finally the stiff-beaten whites. Put all in a well-greased mold or china dish and bake 1 hour. Serve witb the juice of the gooseberries.

NUT PUDDING.

Thirty fresh peanuts or walnuts grated without being blanched; then add 6 ounces of bread or zwieback soaked in milk and drained; cream the butter with the yolks of the eggs, sugar and ½ cup of sweet cream. Mix all thoroughly together, adding then the well-beaten whites of the eggs, and bake in a greased pudding dish for 1 hour and serve with foam sauce. For 8 or 10 persons.

SOUR CREAM PUDDING.

Take 1 quart of sour cream, 6 or 8 eggs, 3 or 4 spoonfuls of flour, sugar, vanilla and a little salt. Beat the cream well, then add the other ingredients, and finally the stiff-beaten whites of the eggs, and bake for 45 minutes. For 6 or 8 persons.

PECAN PUDDING.

Beat 1 tablespoonful of butter to a cream; add 2 tablespoonfuls of sugar, 3 ounces stale white bread (soaked in water and drained), yolks of 6 eggs and 30 or 40 grated pecan nuts; finally, stir in the stiff-beaten whites of the eggs and bake the pudding for 1 hour in a well-greased mold. Serve with fruit juice.

COLD PUDDINGS AND CREAMS.

RED GRITS.

Take 1 pint of raspberry juice, 1 pint of water, 3 ounces grits or sago and sugar to taste.

Cook the sugar and juice together till done, but not too stiff; then wet a china dish with cold water and pour all into it. When cold, turn out into a large plate and serve with vanilla cream and sugar well beaten together.

RICE CREAM.

Boil ½ pound best rice in 1 quart of sweet cream with grated peel of ½ lemon. Beat ¼ pound of sugar with the juice of 3 lemons, boil till stiff and stir into the cooked rice (take off from the fire); soak 1 ounce red gelatine in warm water and add it to the other ingredients. Arrange this with canned or fine cooked fruit in a dish in layers. Let it cool till stiff, then turn out on a platter and garnish with fruits.

RED FLAMMERY.

Five cups of sweet milk, 3 ounces of sugar, 3 ounces of bitter almonds and 3 ounces of sweet almonds grated, a little vanilla or lemon peel and 1 ounce of red gelatine.

Boil the first four ingredients together; add the gelatine, which has been soaked in warm water; rinse a dish out with cold water without drying it, and pour all into it to get cold. Serve with fruit juice.

LEMON CREAM.

Bring ¾ of a quart of water with 6 ounces of sugar to a boil; add grated peel of 1 lemon, juice of 3 lemons, yolks of 6 eggs, 2 tablespoonfuls of corn-starch dissolved in water, and boil till done, stirring constantly. Take off and let it cool, then mix with the stiff-beaten whites of the eggs; put in a dish to get cold; turn out and serve with fruit juice. For 10 persons.

CHOCOLATE CREAM.

Six ounces sweet chocolate, 6 eggs, 4 ounces sugar, a little vanilla and ½ ounce gelatine.

Melt the chocolate over the fire in a little water; take off and add to it, while stirring, the sugar and vanilla, and then the yolks of the eggs; beat all together well, put back on the fire and let cook till it comes to a boil; then set aside and add the gelatine dissolved in water and the stiff-beaten whites of the eggs. Put it in a china dish wet with cold water. When ready to serve turn out and serve with beaten sweet cream.

CREAM WITH ALMONDS.

One pint of good fresh cream, 2 ounces finely grated almonds, ½ pound sugar.

Cook all 15 minutes and let cool, then beat 4 eggs and the yolks of 3 eggs into it. Pour this mixture into custard cups and set them in hot water to thicken. If to be served cold set on ice.

TUTTI-FRUTTI.

Cover the bottom of a large glass dish with macaroons and lady-fingers; pour over this fruit juice and unfermented grape juice to taste, and let soak 1 hour. Meanwhile let come to a boil 1 tablespoonful of butter, to which add 3 pints of milk and the yolks of 5 large eggs; add sugar and vanilla to taste; stir till thick, but do not let it come to a boil; take off, let it cool and pour over the cakes in the dish. Beat the whites of the eggs stiff, sweeten with sugar and fruit jelly and spread on top.

CREAM OF CORN-STARCH.

One and one-eighth quarts of water, ¼ pound of sugar, ¼ pound corn-starch or corn-meal, juice of 3 lemons and grated peel of 1.

Let the lemon juice, peel, sugar and half of the water come to a boil. Mix the corn-starch in the other half of the water and add to the other ingredients; boil for 10 minutes. Serve with any kind of fruit sauce.

ORANGE CREAM.

Beat 1 quart of sweet cream, juice of 6 or 8 oranges and ½ pound of sugar. Beat all well together, then add 1 ounce of dissolved gelatine and serve in a glass dish.

GOOSEBERRY DISH.

One quart of green gooseberries, cleaned and washed; boil them with 1 quart of water till done; stir through a sieve, and sweeten. Put on the fire and stir into it ½ pound of rice flour, which is mixed with the gooseberry juice. Let it boil for awhile, stirring all the time; then pour into a dish wet with cold water and serve with sweet cream.

SAGO PUDDING.

Soak ¼ pound sago in hot water; pour off the water and add ½ pint of raspberry and ½ pint of currant juice, with sugar and lemon juice to taste; boil till stiff, being careful not to let burn. Serve with cream or milk.

STRAWBERRY CREAM.

Two pounds ripe strawberries, ½ pound of sugar, whites of 6 eggs, 1 glass of cider or unfermented grape juice.

Wash the berries well, pour the water off of them and then stir through a sieve. Boil the grape juice with the sugar; add the fruit and a tablespoonful of corn-starch; stir frequently till it comes to a boil again; take off, beat the whites of the eggs stiff and stir into the fruit. Serve garnished with fine ripe strawberries.

DELICIOUS FRUIT DISH.

Cut 2 bananas in fine lengthwise slices and lay them in a glass dish, upon this a layer of a ripe pineapple cut in small pieces, and then a layer of sliced oranges; pour sugar and a little water over and continue these layers of bananas, oranges and pineapples till the dish is full. If canned pineapple is used, take the juice instead of the water. Put on ice. A delicious desert for hot days.

RASPBERRY FOAM.

Beat the whites of 5 eggs very stiff and stir into it 3 tablespoonfuls of raspberry jelly and ½ tablespoonful of sugar. Serve in glasses.

APPLE CREAM.

Cook one soup-plate of sliced apples in plenty of sugar; cover the bottom of a glass dish with them; over this put a layer of biscuit cakes 2 inches deep. Meanwhile let 1 quart of milk come to a boil with a little vanilla, into which pour a tablespoonful of corn-starch dissolved in a little milk; boil, stirring all the while. Finally, add the well-beaten yolks of 3 eggs and pour over the apples and biscuits. After it is cool, add the beaten whites and garnish with jelly.

VANILLA CREAM.

Five pints of milk, 6 eggs, 1 tablespoonful of corn-starch, sugar to taste and add a little vanilla.

Put all together in a clean cooking vessel over the fire and just before it comes to a boil take off, beat a little and put in a glass dish. Serve with fruit juice.

LEMON JELLY.

Take 3 pints of water, the juice of 6 or 8 lemons, 5 ounces of sugar, 2 tablespoonfuls of corn-starch or best flour dissolved in a little of the water, yolks of 6 eggs well beaten, the grated peel of 1 lemon; boil all together till stiff, take off, and when done add the whites of the eggs beaten stiff, and serve with sweet milk and sweet crackers, or garnished with fruit jelly.

Instead of 6 or 8 lemons, take ½ bottle of unfermented grape juice and the juice of 2 lemons. In case one does not wish to use the grape juice and the 6 or 8 lemons, these may be omittted, using all the other ingredients, and finally mixing 3 tablespoonfuls of currant or raspberry jelly, to give a pretty color and taste.

PUECKLER ICE CREAM.

Whip cream till it is stiff and sweeten as for ice cream. Divide this in thirds; flavor the first third with vanilla; the second color pink with raspberry juice and the third color with chocolate, first having dissolved the chocolate in a very little milk. Mix into each part a few macaroons.

Put in an ice-cream freezer in layers; do not turn nor stir; let it stand a day or longer, if necessary, to freeze, keeping covered with ice.

DRINKS.

ALMOND MILK.

Take half a cup of blanched almonds, grate them in a nut grater, pour a cup of cold water over them and let draw 10 minutes; then squeeze through a clean cloth and give to the patient. It must be made fresh every time, as it sours easily.

Almond milk is of the greatest help in questions of nourishment for the patient, because it contains the greatest amount of nourishment in the smallest form, and with the least work to the digestive organs. Therefore we give it in all diseases of the digestive organs, feverish diseases and to weak persons, with the best results.

CARAMEL CEREAL COFFEE.

Take 2 large cups of this coffee and 10 cups of cold water; bring to a boil for 15 minutes.

DR. LAHMANN'S NAEHRSALZ COCOA.

Take for each cup of water 1 teaspoonful of cocoa, 1 teaspoonful of sugar and 1 teaspoonful of corn-starch for every 5 cups.

SOUR MILK.

Put fresh milk into a stone pot, let stand for 1 or 2 days in a room at about 60° F. The skin on top must be light yellow and shiny; before serving stir in cream with the milk well. Put on ice in summer and serve in glasses.

RASPBERRY LEMONADE.

Two quarts of water mixed well with 2 cupfuls of raspberry juice.

LEMONADE.

Take juice of 1 lemon, add 2 tablespoonfuls of sugar and 2 cups of water.

www.ingramcontent.com/pod-product-compliance
Lightning Source LLC
Chambersburg PA
CBHW072355290526
45794CB00001B/77